The Pediatrician's Role in Promoting Health and Safety in Child Care

Developed in conjunction with the Early Brain and Child Development Initiative, a partnership effort
of the American Academy of Pediatrics and the Johnson & Johnson Pediatric Institute

Johnson&Johnson pediatricinstitute
Division of Johnson & Johnson Consumer Companies, Inc.

Library of Congress Control Number: 2001135191

ISBN: 1-58110-076-0

MA0175

The recommendations in this publication do not indicate an exclusive course of treatment or serve as
a standard of medical care. Variations, taking into account individual circumstances, may be appropriate.

Table of Contents

Preface

Why Do Pediatricians Need to Be Involved in Child Care?

When the famous bank robber, Willie Sutton, was asked why he robbed banks, he replied, "Because that's where the money is." So why, then, do pediatricians need to be involved in child care? Because that's where the children are: Nearly 75% of children under 5 years of age, including 50% of infants, attend some type of child care on a regular basis. The proportion of children in child care has doubled over the past 30 years as more parents return to work and school.[1]

Over the past few decades, a considerable amount of research has examined outcomes for children in child care compared to children cared for at home. Overall, studies have found that children in child care are at greater risk for infectious diseases but at no increased risk for attachment difficulties, delays in socio-emotional or cognitive development, injuries, or child abuse. In contrast, studies have found that children in high-quality child care may have significant advantages in socio-emotional and cognitive development. Over the years, the discourse on child care has shifted from examining the risks to identifying the opportunities that quality child care can provide children and families.[2]

Recent discoveries about early brain and child development underscore the importance of high-quality child care. "The human brain is relatively undeveloped at birth, its potential waiting to unfold as its structure takes shape, and depends upon individual experience to guide its growth," writes Edward L. Schor, MD, FAAP, in the book *Early Brain Development and Child Care.* "Experiences and sensory inputs (visual, auditory, tactile, olfactory, and taste) organize patterns of communication between neurons. These neural patterns become the determinants of how we think, feel, and behave."[3] There are "windows of opportunity" and "prime times," that occur during the first 3 years of life, during which the child's brain is most effective in processing experiences. Research has demonstrated that consistent, warm, and responsive relationships and a stimulating learning environment in early childhood are crucial to promote children's early development and lay the foundation for socio-emotional and cognitive skills for life.[4]

Since most young children spend a significant amount of time in child care, the quality of children's relationships with their caregivers and the child care environment have a tremendous impact on children's development, health, safety, and overall well-being.

Studies of child care programs in the United States, however, have shown that the quality of care ranges from excellent to poor, and the majority of young children receive "mediocre" care that may compromise their development, health, and safety.[5, 6]

Pediatricians can play a vital role in promoting children's health and well-being by becoming passionate advocates for quality child care. With your trusting relationship with families and frequent contact during children's early years, you can make a difference by counseling families on how to find the child care that is best for their child. With your respected role in the community, you also can help improve health and safety standards in child care by providing health consultation to community child care programs.

How Are Pediatricians Currently Involved in Child Care?

From 1998–1999, the American Academy of Pediatrics (AAP) surveyed pediatricians about their involvement in child care.[7] Nearly three quarters of the pediatricians who responded to the survey believed that it was their role to help improve the quality of child care in their community, and nearly two thirds believed that pediatricians should provide services or consultation to child care programs.

At well-child visits with patients under age 4, 80% of pediatricians routinely inquired about whether the child was in child care and 70% inquired about the type of child care setting. Only 30% of pediatricians, however, routinely discussed child care during prenatal counseling. While two thirds of pediatricians routinely initiated discussion about returning to work after childbirth, continuing breastfeeding while working, and deciding when a child could return to child care after an illness, fewer than one fourth of pediatricians routinely discussed child care issues with parents. However, parents may look to their pediatricians hoping to discuss how to evaluate the quality of child care settings, how to choose the optimum child care environment for their child, options for when a child is too ill to attend child care, and dealing with behavioral problems in child care. Unfortunately, fewer than 1 in 6 pediatricians were reported to be actively involved with local child care programs by providing health consultation or educational sessions on health and safety issues for child care providers.

Pediatricians cited numerous reasons why they were significantly less involved in child care than they believed was important. Two thirds of pediatricians said they did not know how to get involved. Nearly two thirds said that they lacked knowledge about child care issues. Nine out of 10 pediatricians had no education on child care issues during medical school or residency, three fourths had not attended any continuing medical education (CME) or grand rounds programs on child care issues, and more than half had not read any journal articles or books on health in child care. More than two thirds were unaware of key resources available on health and safety in child care. In all, however, 6 out of 10 pediatricians were interested in information about how they could become more involved in child care.

The American Academy of Pediatrics supports the role that pediatricians can play in the child care setting. The AAP policy statement, *Universal Access to Good-quality Education and Care of Children From Birth to 5 Years,* states that to promote optimal child health and development, pediatricians should work not only with parents, but also with other caregivers, agencies, and organizations that are part of the child's and family's support system. The AAP also believes that pediatricians have the education and expertise to potentially protect hundreds or thousands of children. In addition, the AAP is prepared to support pediatrician involvement in child care through technical assistance, resources, and support through its publications, and the federally funded Healthy Child Care America campaign.

How Are You Involved in Child Care?

Take this opportunity to examine how involved *you* are in promoting children's health in child care. Think about how confident you are in your ability to
- Help parents understand their child's developmental and health needs, and how to find the child care that is best for their child.

- Explain to parents the differences between in-home care, family child care, and child care centers; between licensed and unlicensed care; and between preschool and Head Start programs.
- Tell parents where they can get referrals for child care programs in their community.
- Advise parents what to look for in quality infant, toddler, and preschool programs.
- Give parents suggestions for easing the transition to child care.
- Tell parents which illnesses require exclusion from child care and for how many days.
- Develop a plan for caring for children with chronic conditions in child care.
- Explain to caregivers the specific standards for child care health policies.
- Conduct an on-site health and safety check at a child care facility.
- Provide hands-on training on health for child care professionals.
- Advocate for improved health and safety standards for child care in your state.
- Identify national, state, and local resources for information, policies, and referrals.

What Is the Purpose of This Curriculum?

This curriculum is a resource guide designed to help pediatricians become more involved in child care issues to promote children's development, health, and safety. It contains practical information and materials to help you work with families and child care providers in many different ways. While it is oriented toward primary care pediatricians, it also contains issues that are relevant to pediatric subspecialists caring for children who may attend child care.

The curriculum provides suggestions on how you can be involved in child care on different levels, depending on your interest and time available:
- *Level One: Providing Guidance to Families on Child Care Issues*
  This section offers tips on incorporating child care issues into the individual clinical services that you currently provide. It should be helpful for all practicing pediatricians and requires very little extra time and effort to implement.

⁑ *Level Two: Providing Health Consultation to Child Care Programs*

This section details how to reach out to provide health consultation to local child care programs. It is for pediatricians who are interested in providing community-based services and establishing an ongoing relationship with a child care program to promote health and safety.

⁑ *Level Three: Advocating for Quality Child Care*

This section illustrates how you can take the extra step to promote quality child care in your community and beyond. It is for pediatricians who have a particular interest in community outreach, education, and advocacy.

We encourage you to review the curriculum and the background information on child care. Try out some of the suggestions, and use or modify some of the materials to meet the needs of your practice. Reach out and talk with families about child care, collaborate with local child care providers, and utilize local child care resources. Remember that the first few years of life are crucial for children's health and development. By promoting health and safety in child care, you can make a significant difference in the lives of children and families in your community.

This curriculum was developed by the AAP Division of Community Health Services, the Healthy Child Care America Campaign, and the AAP Committee on Early Childhood, Adoption, and Dependent Care, with funding from Johnson & Johnson Pediatric Institute as part of the AAP Initiative on Early Brain Development. The AAP would like to acknowledge the contributions of the author, Karen Sokal-Gutierrez, MD, MPH, and further thank members of the AAP Committee on Early Childhood, Adoption, and Dependent Care and other numerous pediatricians, child care providers, and parents across the country who provided valuable input.

References

1. US National Center for Health Statistics. *The Monthly Vital Statistics Report.* Washington, DC: The Bureau of the Census; 1996

2. American Academy of Pediatrics. *Health in Child Care: A Manual for Health Professionals.* Elk Grove Village, IL: American Academy of Pediatrics. In press

3. Schor EL. Early brain development and child care. *Healthy Child Care America.* January 1999;3:1, 6–8

4. Shore R. *Rethinking the Brain: New Insights into Early Development.* New York, NY: Families and Work Institute; 1997

5. Heilburn S, Culkin ML. *Cost, Quality and Child Outcomes in Child Care Centers.* Denver, CO: University of Colorado; 1995

6. Galinsky E. *The Study of Children in Family Child Care and Relative Care.* New York, NY: Families and Work Institute; 1994

7. American Academy of Pediatrics. Periodic survey of fellows #41. Pediatricians' experiences with child care health and safety. Available at: http://www.aap.org/research/ps41exs. htm. Accessed September 13, 2001

Level One

Providing Guidance to Families on Child Care Issues

Having a baby can be physically and emotionally challenging for parents. With a newborn baby, a parent's primary concern is usually, "Will I be able to care for my baby's needs?" After a few weeks, however, the parents have become familiar with the baby's rhythms and usually feel more confident caring for their baby. But for parents who are returning to work, the next greatest concern is, "Can I trust *someone else* to care for my baby's needs?"

It is understandable that parents are concerned with child care decisions. Research has shown that adequate care and stimulation in early childhood is crucial for a child's development.[1] Parents' choice of child care can have a tremendous impact on their child's health, development, and well-being. Quality care can benefit a child's development, while poor care has been proven detrimental to children. Unfortunately, studies have found that a significant proportion of child care programs may compromise children's development, health, and safety.[2, 3]

Talk with all your patients about the importance of safe and nurturing child care. Tell parents that you will join in a 3-way partnership—family, pediatrician, and child care provider—to support their child's health and development. Do not lose the opportunity to make a significant difference in the lives of young children and their families.

Prenatal and Well-Child Care Visits

Helping Families Make Decisions About Child Care

Most parents hear about child care programs from a friend or relative, and they make the decision based on cost, location, and available hours. Parents rarely have specific information about how to choose quality child care that promotes their child's development, health, and safety. A recent survey found that only 1% of families found their child care provider through the assistance of their pediatrician.[4]

Finding the right child care is one of the most important and challenging decisions that parents make in caring for their young child. The prenatal visit is the best time to begin discussing child care for the baby. Pediatricians can help parents find child care programs where the child's safety and health are appropriately supported. Parents can benefit from more guidance and support. Pediatricians are a trusted source of guidance for families about the care of their children. You can play a vital role in helping parents make important decisions about child care.

When to Talk With Families About Child Care

Pediatricians can address child care issues at all types of clinical visits—the earlier and more frequently, the better. National guidelines for health supervision recommend that child care be part of "anticipatory guidance" at all well-child visits, beginning with the prenatal visit.[5]

Many parents return to work or school when their infant is 6 to 12 weeks old. Since it can take months for parents to research child care options, interview caregivers, visit programs, and make decisions about child care, the prenatal visit is the best time to begin discussing child care for the baby.

When Tracy and Jeff were in the sixth month of pregnancy with their first child, they saw Mary Jones, MD, a pediatrician in Berkeley, CA, for a prenatal visit. Tracy said, "Dr Jones asked us lots of questions about our family, the pregnancy, and our child care plans. We discussed our search for child care and what we were looking for. If we decided on the nanny, she urged us to get her checked through the child abuse registry. If we decided on the child care center, she explained that the baby would be exposed to more germs and might have frequent illnesses in the first year. But she promised to work with us to make sure the baby's child care situation was the right one. I was really encouraged by her knowledge and support. It was clear that she cared not only about my baby's physical health but also his emotional well-being and ours as well."

Opening Up the Conversation About Child Care

You can introduce child care issues to parents in your waiting room. You may hang a poster on the wall, arrange a bulletin board display, or provide educational brochures and handouts for parents on child care. For example, the AAP brochure, "Child Care: What's Best for Your Family," gives parents an excellent introduction to the different types of child care, what to look for in child care, what to ask the caregiver, child care issues for children at different ages, and tips for preparing for child care. Check with your local child care resource and referral agency for posters and other information that could be informative in directing parents to specific support services.

The Healthy Child Care North Carolina Project developed an attractive poster entitled, "Choosing Child Care." The North Carolina Pediatric Society collaborated to encourage pediatricians to display the poster in their offices. Jim Poole, MD, of Raleigh, NC, member of the Committee on Early Childhood, Adoption, and Dependent Care, said, "The poster catches parents' attention and gets us talking more about child care."

The Pediatric Medical Group of Berkeley, CA, has a notebook in the waiting room with parents' comments about child care programs their children have attended. A parent said, "I read in the child care notebook about some smaller centers and family child care homes that I hadn't known about but sounded great. It's helpful to hear the parents' perspective. And it gives me ideas about programs to visit and what I might look for."

Susan Aronson, MD, of Philadelphia, PA, founder of the Pennsylvania AAP Chapter project, the Early Childhood Education Linkage System (ECELS) said, "I've thought for years that our anticipatory guidance around child care should be like our anticipatory guidance for injury prevention—something at every well-child visit—and we could develop counseling guidelines like the AAP Injury Prevention Program (TIPP)." Dr Aronson developed a 1-page questionnaire entitled "Child (day) Care and Education." Parents complete the questionnaire in her waiting room and then she follows up on their concerns and questions during the well-child visit. (See Child Care Resources: A Pediatrician's Guide to Child Care Consultation.) She says, "This has really helped to open up the conversation about child care."

Parents want to talk with their pediatrician about their child care concerns. They also may need more extensive information than an office assistant, nurse, or health educator can provide. Your office might consider hiring an early childhood specialist with training in child development and experience in coordinating child care programs. An early childhood specialist could assist parents in finding quality child care and address ongoing concerns about child care and developmental and behavioral issues. A recent study found that most parents felt their child's physician provided overall excellent pediatric care, but the majority said they could still use more information on newborn care, sleep patterns, responding to a crying baby, toilet training, discipline, and encouraging early learning.[6] An early childhood specialist could be an invaluable member of your clinical team to help you meet parents' and children's needs.

Talking With Parents About Child Care

Stay informed: Read about child care. Talk with people about child care. Visit different types of child care programs (eg, an infant center, family child care, and Head Start program) to become familiar with their different characteristics. Observe and talk with caregivers about their experiences and concerns with health and safety. The more you know about child care, the more helpful you can be to patients.

Siobhan McNally, MD, of Lenox, MA, says, "I try to ask my patients, colleagues, and friends about the child care their children receive. I like to hear about their experiences with different types of child care programs, particularly how the programs worked with children of different ages, temperaments, and special needs. It's helped me become familiar with the local child care programs and be more helpful to families around their child care concerns."

A preschool teacher noted, "I'd like every pediatrician to have the opportunity to visit an early childhood program regularly. They'd have the chance to observe healthy, normal children at work and play. And they'd see all that we do to promote children's health—handwashing, nutritious meals, toothbrushing, cleaning and disinfecting; and all that we do to support parents' well-being. I think visiting us would help pediatricians gain a greater respect for what we do and feel more eager to work with us."

Open up the topic: Make it a routine part of your prenatal and well-child visits to discuss child care. Use open-ended, nonjudgmental questions such as, "What can you tell me about your plans for child care?" "Do you plan to return to work? To school?" "Have you thought about child care arrangements?" "Are you working outside your home or going to school?" "Who helps you care for (child's name)?" Asking nonjudgmental questions about the parents' plans for child care assumes that some child care will be needed, if only for adult activities of the parents individually or together as a couple. Ask the parents about their thoughts, experiences, concerns, and questions about the child care they are using. Expect that parents are using multiple caregivers for different situations.

Help parents weigh their child care considerations: Each child and family has unique characteristics, desires, and needs. No single decision about child care is right for every child and family. Parents must weigh the considerations for their own child and their own circumstances.

* Will they stay home with their child or use child care?
* At what age will they start child care?
* How many hours of child care will they use?
* What type of child care will they choose?

Underscore the importance of quality child care: Discuss with parents how consistent, warm, and responsive care for their young child lays an important foundation for the child's healthy development. Reassure parents that the effort they put into finding good child care can benefit their child immensely.

"I've heard some pediatricians praising the advantages of group care for early childhood development—socialization, intellectual development, exposure to different personalities and cultures. It warms my heart when it's acknowledged that we're doing good things for children and families." (Child care provider)

Be supportive: Child care can be a very sensitive issue for parents. They may feel torn between a desire to stay home with their child and a need to return to work or school, or between a desire to return to work or school and pressure from family members or friends to stay home to provide child care. Be nonjudgmental and understanding of parents' concerns. Since parents and child care staff provide early brain stimulation to children, parents who remain at home must also receive support and guidance about how best to assist in their child's development. Respect the fact that families rely on child care to meet their financial, professional, and personal needs. While the combination of work and family life may stress the family, it offers rewards in self-esteem for the parents from the world of adults and gives children models for adult work roles with a gender balance that fits the parents' values. The right balance of work and family life is a very personal decision. Parents appreciate help from trusted advisors to figure out what amount of work and family life is most comfortable for them at any particular stage in their lives.

"I was happy that my pediatrician understood and accepted that I had to work and that my baby would need outside child care. He gave me the support, validation, and help that I needed." (Parent)

Explain that different types of child care have different characteristics, advantages, and disadvantages. (See Child Care Resources: General Child Care Information, and "Child Care: What's Best for Your Family?".) Families choose among the child care options based on their individual preference and finding the right match with their child's particular needs. In addition, they need to weigh the family's concerns for sibling care, convenient hours and location, reliability, flexibility, and cost of care.

Help parents understand how a particular type of child care might be best suited to their child's developmental stage, temperament, and special health or developmental needs. For example,

* An infant with a history of chronic otitis media, a premature infant with severe bronchopulmonary dysplasia, or a child with Acquired Immunodeficiency Syndrome (AIDS) and significant immunosuppression might be better suited in an in-home or small family child care setting with limited exposure to infectious diseases.
* A 2-year-old who is temperamentally sensitive, shy, or highly distractible might do better in a family child care home or a center with small groups and high adult-child ratios.
* A 3-year-old who is very social and physically active might do well in a child care center, preschool, or family child care with a large indoor and outdoor space.

Jody Murph, MD, member of the AAP Committee on Early Childhood, Adoption, and Dependent Care, and a pediatric infectious disease specialist in Iowa City, IA, says, "We're seeing more and more children with special needs in their health, development, and behavior. It's crucial that we help families understand their children's needs and find the child care program that best promotes their child's development, health, and safety."

Provide information on finding child care: Give parents guidance, written information, and referrals to help them find child care. Encourage parents to follow the steps outlined in the brochures on choosing child care (see Child Care Resources: Caring for Your Child: Making the Right Choice). Encourage parents to do the following:

※ Consult with child care resource organizations. For example, every area in the United States has a local child care resource and referral agency that can provide information for parents describing how to select quality child care programs and local child care options. The state child care licensing agency lists facilities that are licensed and regulated and meet minimum quality standards. The National Association for the Education of Young Children (NAEYC) and the National Association for Family Child Care (NAFCC) list child care programs that have earned accreditation requiring higher standards. There are many other organizations, books, and Web sites with helpful information on child care for parents. (See Child Care Resources.)

※ Talk about child care options with family members, friends, and neighbors.

※ Identify several possible child care options that appear satisfactory.

※ Interview the caregivers about their training in early childhood development, health and safety, and their approach to nutrition, toilet training, discipline, parent involvement, etc.

※ Visit each child care program long enough to closely observe how happy the children appear; how caring, warm, and responsive the caregivers are with children and adults; and whether the caregiver follows hygiene and safety precautions. Count the number of caregivers and children to ensure that the group is small enough and there are enough caregivers to provide individualized attention to children. Observe the facilities to ensure that there are appropriate toys, safe play areas indoors and outdoors, and adequate hygiene (especially hand washing and sanitary diaper changing routines).

※ Request references of several families whose children have attended the child care program. Call them and ask them about their experiences with the caregiver.

※ Double-check for safety: Check the licensing agency for complaints against the caregiver or child care program. Request that the caregiver complete a safety check through the state registry for child abuse.

※ Select a child care program that appears to have good quality and the right fit for the child and family.

※ Once their child starts with a new caregiver, plan a trial period in which they observe closely how things are going.

Bruce Gach, MD, chairperson, AAP California Chapter 1, Committee on Early Childhood, Adoption, and Dependent Care, says, "There's so much information out there about child care—I always refer families to the child care resource and referral agency. I keep the child care resource and referral agency number handy next to the telephone in each exam room."

Remind parents to consider back-up child care arrangements for when their child is ill: Don't forget to discuss the fact that young children may experience frequent illnesses, especially in the first year of child care. Although the frequent illnesses can be difficult for children and families, reassure parents that the illnesses can help develop children's immunity and protect them in the future. Discuss with parents the following options for sick-child care:

※ Will their usual caregiver care for their sick child?

※ Will a parent, family member, or friend stay home with the sick child?

※ Will they use a child care program for mildly ill children?

※ Check with state and local health departments for infectious disease policies as they relate to child care, including return to child care policies.

"There's so much to plan with starting child care. I didn't even think about what we'd do when my child got sick. But our pediatrician advised us to have a back-up plan, and a back-up for the back-up. My child got sick after 3 weeks in child care, on a day I had an important meeting. Thank goodness we were prepared." (Parent)

Helping Families Create Partnerships With Their Child's Caregiver

The transition to child care can be challenging for young children, parents, and caregivers alike. Parents and children can have mixed feelings of excitement, anticipation, sadness, and fear. Parents also may have mixed feelings about the practical details of returning to work or school and starting child care. Pediatricians can play an important role in helping families prepare for child care and providing support to ease the transition.

Document the child care program in the child's medical chart: Devote a place on the history form or add a sticker to the chart with the name and telephone number of the child care program. In addition, a parent questionnaire was developed by Dr Aronson to assist pediatricians in identifying child care programs that are being used by their patients. This questionnaire also can assist the families in discussing pertinent child care issues with their primary care provider. (See Child Care Resources: A Pediatrician's Guide to Child Care Consultation.)

Complete the admission requirements: Make sure the child is up-to-date on immunizations and health screenings. Ask the parent to bring the health forms required by the child care program—which may require documentation of health history, physical examination, hearing/vision screening, immunizations, and standing orders for sunscreen or medications. Complete the necessary health forms for child care so caregivers have your detailed instructions and know whom to contact if they have questions.

Develop individual care plans for children with special needs: If the child has special health or developmental needs, discuss with parents the importance of sharing information and working together with the caregiver to meet the child's needs. Some parents may not understand the importance of discussing the child's asthma when the child has had only a couple of asthma attacks each year, or they may be afraid to discuss their

child's behavioral difficulties or Human Immuno-deficiency virus (HIV) infection for fear of discrimination. Explain that the 3-way partnership—among family, pediatrician, and caregiver—is key to ensuring their child's optimal health and development. Work with the parents and caregiver to develop a written care plan for each child who may have special needs and will be enrolled in a child care program. (See Child Care Resources: Sample Individualized Health Plan.)

Ask parents about their concerns and their plans for the transition to child care: Be understanding and supportive. According to the 1999 AAP Periodic Survey #41, *Pediatricians' Experiences with Child Care Health and Safety,* only one quarter of pediatricians initiate child care discussions.[7] Following are several suggestions that pediatricians can use to begin conversations with parents to help ease the transition into child care:

- **Breastfeeding.** Is the baby breastfeeding? Does the mother want to continue breastfeeding? Remind mothers that it is possible and healthy to continue breastfeeding during mornings, evenings, and weekends when the baby is not in child care. When the baby is away from the mother, the baby can be fed expressed breast milk or formula. Maintaining routines, such as breastfeeding, can enhance the baby's comfort and ease the transition to child care. Suggest that parents start giving the baby a bottle (formula or breast milk) every few days at least a couple of weeks before the transition to child care so the baby learns to feed from the bottle. This will help make feeding comfortable with the caregiver. Discuss the considerations for breast milk versus formula, and guidelines for pumping and storing breast milk. (See Child Care Resources: "Supporting Breastfeeding Mothers as They Return to Work.") The AAP pamphlet, "A Woman's Guide to Breastfeeding," can be referenced for additional information.[8]

"In my infant room, I've taken care of many breast-fed babies that just start to take a bottle when they started child care. It can be heartbreaking to care for them through the simultaneous transition to a new caregiver and to the bottle. Pediatricians can really be helpful when they advise parents to begin the bottle at home so babies are comfortable with it when they start child care." (Caregiver)

❖ **Communication.** Encourage parents to talk with their child about the new child care program in the weeks before starting. Being prepared helps young children feel in control and comfortable. Toddlers and preschoolers typically become excited about starting school and becoming "a big boy" or "big girl." Suggest that parents read books that show what child care and preschool is like. They can explain to the child about activities in child care, playing with toys, climbing on the playground, singing, eating lunch, and taking a nap. Remind parents to discuss child care in small doses, gauging their child's reaction, and being careful not to overwhelm or frighten their child.

❖ **Build Relationships.** Suggest that parents take their child to visit the child care program and stay with the child and caregiver several times before leaving the child with the caregiver. The child will become more comfortable with the new caregiver and environment when the parent is present.

❖ **Information.** Urge parents to talk with the caregiver about their child's development, temperament, routines, special needs, and likes and dislikes. The more caregivers know about the child, the better care they can provide.

❖ **Scheduling.** Advise parents to try to ease into the new schedule. If the child will be in full-day care, they might try to start with shorter hours for several days. If they return to the full-time schedule on a Wednesday or Thursday, they can start out with a 2- or 3-day week the first week of work.

❖ **Security.** Remind parents that a "transitional object," such as a picture, stuffed animal, or blanket, can help ease the transition to child care. They should discuss this issue with the caregiver to ensure a common approach.

❖ **Consistency.** Urge parents to establish consistent, reliable routines. They should make an effort to drop off and pick up the child on time. If they plan a different schedule on a particular day, they should tell the child in advance, "Today you're staying a little longer at school and daddy will pick you up after the afternoon snack time instead."

❖ **Timing.** Advise parents to try to avoid the pressure to rush at the morning drop-off and evening pick-up at child care and try to take the time for a relaxed transition. They might develop a special ritual with a favorite toy, a hug, or a kiss. In the morning, when children see their parents talking comfortably with the caregiver and acting confident when saying goodbye, it helps them feel comfortable staying with the caregiver. And at the end of the day when the parents spend time talking with the caregiver about their children's day, and allowing the children to complete their activity and show their parents what they did, it helps them feel valued.

"I felt so bad when I first dropped off my baby in child care and she reached out her arms to me and cried and cried. I had such a hard time leaving. And I cried all the way to work. Then I thought it might be better just to sneak out when she wasn't looking. But my caregiver said that she cried worse when she discovered I was gone. She gave me a brochure, "So Many Goodbyes" that explained it was better to be relaxed, let her know I was leaving and tell her when I'd be back. That was really helpful. And now she doesn't cry anymore when it is time for me to leave—I feel so much better about leaving her there." (Parent) The brochure, "So Many Goodbyes," was developed by the National Association for the Education of Young Children. (See Child Care Resources.)

Remind parents of the importance of good communication with the caregiver: Parents and caregivers are partners in raising the child—this is an important relationship to nurture.

Jeree Pawl, PhD, an infant mental health specialist in San Francisco, CA, says, "Do unto others as you would have them do unto others"—Treat the caregiver as you would like them to treat your child, with care and respect.

Encourage parents to do the following:

❖ Ask the caregiver about his or her life and acknowledge them on birthdays and holidays.

❖ Take a minute every day at drop-off and pick-up time to talk about anything significant that happened with their child. Did she have a visit with grandma last night? How is his appetite and sleep? Does she seem to be teething? Is he starting to take steps? Is she beginning to make sentences? Did he play with a new friend? Did she put together a puzzle? Are there any symptoms of illness?

❖ Include the caregiver in special events such as the child's birthday celebration or dance performance. Invite the caregiver home for a visit. However, be respectful of the caregiver's personal time and obligations.

⁂ At least twice a year, schedule time to talk with the caregiver in more detail about their child and any special needs or concerns they may have.

"Rosa cared for my daughter for 3 years. She was fabulous. She was like a second mother for my daughter, a co-mother for me, a part of our family. Every day I so much looked forward to Rosa telling me something wonderful my daughter did that day. I truly feel that a big part of my daughter's love of life came from her great relationship with Rosa." (Parent)

Following Up and Supporting Child Care Programs

Although parents may put a lot of work into selecting the right child care program, that is just the beginning. It takes even more effort to continually nurture the child care relationship, observe how the child is doing, and work out any problems that may arise. The transition to child care can take months. And a child care situation that may have been right for the infant may no longer fit for the toddler or preschooler. The pediatrician can play an important role in routine follow-up and supporting parents' child care concerns at every well-child visit.

Peter Gorski, MD, member of the Committee on Early Childhood, Adoption, and Dependent Care and a developmental specialist in Boston, MA, said, "The research on early brain development shows us that pediatricians must support parents' emotional well-being and family well-being—this is primary to infant attachment and socio-emotional development. We must recognize the importance of relationships and compassion, beginning in the pediatrician-patient relationship."

Address questions and concerns about child care: The transition to child care and work/school can be stressful for children and parents. It is common for children to experience changes with the transition to child care. For example, they may regress in their behavior or have changes in sleep or appetite. They also may experience a "honeymoon period" for a few weeks during which they eagerly accept child care, but then go through a period of angry resistance. Reassure parents that it is normal for children to experience changes during the transition and give them tips on how to talk with their children about their feelings. For example, with a child who refuses to put on her shoes to go to school, a parent could say, "Sometimes you feel like such a big girl at school. And sometimes you still want to be a little girl and have only mom take care of you. That's okay. You put on one shoe and I'll help you with the other."

⁂ Ask about the child: How does he seem to have adjusted to child care? How comfortable does she seem to be with the caregiver? Does he seem happy to go to child care? How is her appetite and sleeping? How is his development progressing? What activities does she enjoy? How is he getting along with other children?

⁂ Ask about the parents: How have they adjusted to returning to work or school? How has their mood and energy level been? How has their relationship been with their child and other family members? How is their relationship with the caregiver?

Update records of the child care situation: Have the office assistant or nurse ask the parent, "Who cares for your child during the day?" Update the chart with any new child care information.

Dr Bruce Gach of Livermore, CA, says, "I always try to touch bases about child care at every visit. Most of what I do is reassure parents that they're doing okay, that their kids are doing okay, that their kids are okay in child care. Kids in child care do get sick—it's okay."

It is also common for parents to experience distress with the transition to child care. A recent survey found that parents said that "the worst thing about child care" was that their child was sick more often. Parents' concern about their children's illness in child care was 3 times higher than the next most common concerns—missing their child and fear that the caregiver didn't provide adequate stimulation for their child.[4] Many parents feel separation anxiety, sadness, or guilt about leaving their child. Some parents feel jealous of the caregiver who gets to cuddle their child during the day or share their child's joy of her first steps and other milestones. Some parents feel pressured to have their child make developmental leaps such as toilet training, learning letters, and numbers. Listen attentively and provide support for parents' feelings.

"When I'd pick up my 2-year-old at child care, the teacher would say he'd been great all day. But then when I tried to get him to leave and get into the car to go home, he'd be kicking and screaming. I felt awful—What was I doing wrong? Why was he so good for them and not for me? But my pediatrician was really helpful—She said it's totally normal— even her own child did it. She said it's a good sign that he was happy all day at school. He's worked so hard to keep it together all day. And it's a good sign that he can let out all his feelings with me because he trusts me. She also suggested a special routine for the drive home. So we started playing his music tapes and that's helped a lot." (Parent)

"At first when I picked up my child in the afternoon, I was upset when she was dirty and her clothes were stained with paint. But our pediatrician asked, 'Is she dirty at the end of the day? That shows she really had a good time.' She helped me see it in another way." (Parent)

"When my child was in preschool, I started wondering why he just played all the time—wasn't he going to learn the ABCs? When I mentioned my concern to the pediatrician, he said, 'The work of preschool is play. Does your child seem happy? Does he enjoy playing with other children, exploring the environment, and trying new activities?' My child was very active and happy at school. It helped me understand what was best for my child's development." (Parent)

Also listen for "red flags" that might indicate a poor fit with the caregiver, neglect, or abuse. Sometimes the first indicator is the parent's sense that "something just isn't right." Encourage parents to talk with you about their concerns and to talk with the caregiver to try to work through the problems. Sometimes it just takes time and a special effort for the child care relationship to develop, especially for children who are temperamentally sensitive or who are 6 to 12 months old and experiencing stranger fear and separation anxiety. But sometimes the "fit" just isn't right and a different child care program might be indicated. Refer families to available resources such as the local child care resource and referral agency or mental health services, if necessary. Follow up sus-

pected child abuse/neglect per protocols. (See Child Care Resources: Child Care Aware contact information.)

"Hannah was happy for several years in family child care, but when she was 3 years old we thought a preschool would be good for her. We visited preschools and found one that seemed perfect— well-trained and nurturing caregivers, developmentally appropriate curriculum, safe facilities. But from the start, Hannah just didn't seem happy there. She started coming home saying 'I don't like it' and 'The kids are scary.' And she became increasingly resistant to going to school every morning. She also became resistant to toileting. We tried to work with the teachers and we kept her there for 4 months, hoping things would get better. But they never did. There was nothing wrong with the program, it just wasn't right for Hannah. I realized that I had to listen to the cues my child was giving me. We placed her back into her family child care and she's been very happy since." (Parent)

"My child is blind now after her caregiver shook her violently when she was an infant. I keep replaying it in my mind, wishing that I could undo it. In retrospect, I think I should've responded to my earliest suspicions that something wasn't right in the way the caregiver interacted with my child. But it was my first child—What did I know? Now I tell everyone I can: Follow your instincts. You can never be too careful with your precious children." (Parent)

Provide anticipatory guidance: When the child is cared for both at home and in child care, the anticipatory guidance should be directed toward parents and caregivers. For example,

- When discussing car seats, seat belts, and air bags, remind parents that they should make sure their children are transported safely on the way to, from, and during child care.
- If you give a handout to parents on child-proofing their home for their infant, you might give them another copy to share with the caregiver.
- When discussing appropriate discipline or toilet training, advise parents to make sure that the caregiver's approach is compatible with theirs.

"I feel the best thing parents can do to prepare their child for child care is to ensure they get a good night's sleep every night. I know that working parents miss their children and keep them up at night to be together. But we really see the fall-out in child care. Pediatricians could help by explaining to parents that a little more sleep really makes a big difference." (Caregiver)

"When I had my third child, my pediatrician gave me the brochure 'Back to Sleep' and discussed the new recommendations for putting babies to sleep. This was new to me. So I thought I should talk with the caregiver about it since she'd had her kids so long ago. She said this was new to her too. But she had a niece that died of Sudden Infant Death Syndrome (SIDS) so she said she really wanted to follow the new recommendations for my baby. I'm glad we talked about it." (Parent)

"I take care of my grandson while my daughter is in school. When I brought him in for his 12-month check-up, the pediatrician said, 'It looks like he's starting to walk well now! Let's make sure you've child-proofed your house. Do you have any medications around that you're taking...?' I hadn't even thought that my grandson might get into my medication on my bedside table, not to mention all the other dangers around my house. He gave me a brochure on child-proofing and I went right home and had my kids help me make my house safe." (Caregiver)

Promote a 3-way partnership among pediatrician, parents, and caregivers: Remind parents that it is best for their child's health and development when you all work together. Explain that sometimes it is helpful for you to share information in writing or talk directly with the caregiver, such as when there are concerns about their child's development or medications. Ask the parent for written consent for you and the child's caregiver/teacher to share information directly, if needed. If you have special hours or special procedures for taking calls from caregivers, give instructions to the parents to share with the caregiver.

The pediatric practice of Tom Tonniges, MD, hosted a child care fair in Nebraska during NAEYC's Week of the Young Child. The practice invited several local child care directors to answer parents' questions about child care and early childhood development. He said, "The child care fair was a nice way to establish a professional alliance with child care providers and offer parents a valuable educational opportunity."

Caring for Children With Acute Conditions

When children attend child care, the child care provider is involved with the family in every aspect of the child's health and development and often serves the role of extended family for the parents. When treatment plans are developed, remember that the caregiver is a key partner in the care of the child. Valuable information about the child's health and development should go both ways—to and from the caregiver.

Obtaining Information From the Parents and Caregiver

Review the information on child's signs and symptoms from the parents and the child care provider: Even though the parent may bring the child into your office for an acute illness or injury, the illness might have developed or the injury might have occurred at child care. Often, the parent is called from work to pick up the child from child care but is not well-informed about the details of the child's condition.

To establish an accurate history of the episode, it is helpful for the caregiver to provide brief, written documentation of the child's condition. The caregiver should complete a Symptom Record or Injury Report and give a copy to the parents to share with you. The Symptom Record or Injury Report should detail the incident that occurred, the child's signs and symptoms, and the care that was given to the child. If the child care provider does not document illnesses and injuries, give parents the sample forms to share with their caregiver. (See Child Care Resources: Symptom Record and Injury Report Form.)

Ask the parents about contributing factors at home and child care: When a child spends a significant amount of time in child care, there may be factors at child care that could contribute to a child's illness or injury. For example:

∷ If a child develops an allergic reaction, remember to ask about the child's exposures at home and at child care.

∷ If a child becomes ill with a rash and fever, you may inquire whether anyone else has had similar symptoms at home or at child care. In making your diagnosis, it could be helpful to know that several children in the child care program were diagnosed with scarlet fever.

∷ If a child breaks a leg falling off of a climbing structure at child care, you may ask the parent what action the parents and caregivers have taken to ensure playground safety. Avoid any implication or blame, but offer helpful guidance for what can be done. Consider giving the parent and caregiver a copy of the AAP video, *Safe Active Play,* to help the caregiver review and improve the safety of the outdoor play area to prevent future injuries. Give the parent the AAP Web site address for more playground safety information and how to locate a certified playground inspector.

Offer to speak with the child care provider, if needed. If you need more information that the parent is unable to provide or if the treatment plan is complex, it can be helpful for you to speak directly with the caregiver. Ask the parent for written consent for you to talk with the caregiver, if needed. If you have special hours or special procedures for taking calls from caregivers, give instructions to the parents to share with the caregiver.

Developing the Treatment Plan With the Parents and Caregiver

Simplify treatment recommendations and medications: If medication is needed to treat an acute illness, try to prescribe medication that is convenient to administer. Giving a child medication can be more difficult for a child care provider than for a parent, due to the number of children in their care at one time. Child care providers must also depend on state laws and policies for administering medication to children while in their care. While giving the medication and documenting the procedure, the caregiver also needs to supervise the other children. To simplify treatment for child care providers, pediatricians and parents should develop a plan together.

∷ If possible, prescribe medication so that minimal dispensing has to be done in the child care setting.

∷ If the child needs to be given medication in child care, instruct the pharmacy to split the medication into 2 bottles—1 for home and 1 for child care—to help prevent missed doses when parents and caregivers forget to transfer the medication at drop-off and pick-up times. If the child requires special supplies or equipment, such as an Epi-Pen, inhaler, or a nebulizer, prescribe an extra set for child care, as per state regulatory policies, and arrange for caregivers to receive training from your office staff or prescribe training for caregivers by home health agency personnel (often covered by insurance).

∷ If there are specific instructions for administering the medication that are not listed on the label, prepare written instructions for both the parents and caregiver. (See Child Care Resources: Medication form.)

"Our center requires a doctor's permission slip for medication. We don't feel comfortable giving Joey cough and cold medicine 'as needed.' We need to know that it's medically necessary, the duration of treatment, the dose, and schedule to provide the best care for the child." (Caregiver)

Discuss when the child can return to child care: When a child experiences an acute illness, injury, or other condition, he or she may need to recover at home for a while. But this question—Does the child need to stay home and for how long?—can create significant tension among child care providers, parents, and pediatricians. It is important to appreciate the concerns on all sides.

Parents are concerned about the health of their child and how to provide the proper care so that the child gets well. In addition, however, parents are often concerned with the difficulty of making last-minute arrangements to care for their sick child. Parents' jobs may be inflexible, not allowing them to take leave to care for their children. When a sick child is sent home, parents may fear jeopardizing their jobs and income by taking time off to stay home, or they may need to remain at their jobs and fear jeopardizing the safety of their child by keeping school-age siblings home as caregivers or leaving the child with any available adult.

The caregiver is concerned about the health of the ill child—how to provide the extra attention and care the child might need to get well. The caregiver also is concerned about the health and safety of the other children and staff in the program—how to protect them from catching the illness and continue to give them the attention and care they need.

Pediatricians should address parents' and caregivers' concerns about children's illnesses in a sensitive manner.

∷ Reassure parents and caregivers that frequent illnesses are common in child care, especially in the first year the child attends.

∷ Try not to make parents or caregivers feel guilty for the child's illness.

∷ Remind parents and caregivers of the importance of rest and nurturing to help the child recover, and good hand washing to reduce the spread of the illness to others.

∷ Be understanding of parents' need to return to work or school. Be aware of sick-child care options; discuss and emphasize the importance of having back-up caregivers (eg, family members, friends, neighbors, or a child care facility for ill children) who will care for the child when the child is too sick to attend the regular child care program.

"When I brought my child in for an illness, the doctor said, 'Well, your child's in child care—it's a germ haven.' I already feel awful about my child being sick and feel guilty about having to work and not seeing my child as much as I'd like. What I really need is support." (Parent)

"My pediatrician told me to expect that my children would get sick in child care, but then they'd develop immunity. It was really hard with both my children sick so much that first year in child care. But I found that if we could just hang in through the first winter, then they were healthy after that. The pediatrician was right—she helped me see the light at the end of the tunnel." (Parent)

Above all, be sure to follow the standards for exclusion/readmission for illness that are outlined in the newest edition of the AAP *Red Book: Report of the Committee on Infectious Diseases,*[9] and the AAP/APHA manual, *Caring for Our Children: National Health and Safety Performance Standards: Guidelines for Out-of-Home*

Child Care.[10] These guidelines are also summarized in a booklet called *Preparing for Illness,*[11] available from the AAP. In addition, each state regulates exclusion criteria for licensed child care facilities. For a list of your state's requirements, or to see any of these documents, see Child Care Resources.

The basic criteria for determining when a child is ready to return to child care are as follows:

∷ The child must be well enough to participate comfortably in the program's activities.

∷ The staff must be able to care for the child's needs without compromising the care of other children.

∷ The child must not pose a significant risk for transmission of specific communicable diseases.

The national child care health and safety standards detail the symptoms for which a child should be excluded (eg, fever accompanied by behavior change or other symptoms) and the number of days of exclusion recommended for specific infectious diseases. Ultimately, however, most decisions about whether the child can attend child care are based on the caregiver's policy and judgment about whether the child is well enough to participate and whether the staff can safely care for the child's needs. For example, even though a child may be past the most infectious period of an illness, if the child still needs a lot of rest, the caregiver might determine that the child cannot be cared for because a significant part of the program is outdoor play or a field trip is planned for that day. Remind parents of the importance of respecting the caregiver's general health policy and right to decide about when their child is well enough to attend.

"When a child at our center gets sick, we follow the Standards—We tell the parents that their child needs to be past the contagious period and feel well enough to return to child care. The doctor said, 'Since everyone at child care has already been exposed, she can return to child care.' But the child was still too sick to participate. I'd like doctors to tell parents, 'Your child is no longer contagious. But check with your caregiver about whether the child is up to the physical and emotional demands of the activities in child care.' It's best when doctors and child care programs follow the same standards." (Child care center director)

Document the child's condition for the caregiver: The clearer the communication among the pediatrician, parents, and caregivers, the better. If you have diagnosed a communicable disease, consider giving the parent a brief written report for the caregiver stating the diagnosis, whether the child is contagious, and the treatment plan. (See Child Care Resources: Request for Health Care Provider Evaluation.) This information is important to child care providers as they may also be responsible for reporting certain illnesses to the local health department. Caregivers sometimes ask for a permission slip for the child to return to care. Instead of being annoyed by these requests, discuss with the director when the child care program needs more information than the parent can give. This will help reduce unnecessary requests and improve the caregiver's ability to meet the needs of the recovering child.

Caregivers need to know the diagnosis of an infectious disease. Many child care programs post notices to inform parents about their child's exposure to certain infectious diseases. You can give the parent, or fax to the caregiver, a fact sheet on the disease that can inform parents and caregivers about the disease—how it is spread, the contagious period, the symptoms to look for, how it is diagnosed, whether the child needs to stay home from child care, and how to prevent further spread.

"It's extremely helpful when pediatricians send our child care program a note about the child's illness and what we should do. It helps us be more informed and care for the child better. And it also helps us be more prepared to handle the next illness." (Child care provider)

Report specified conditions to the necessary authorities: State law requires pediatricians and child care providers to report certain communicable diseases and suspected child abuse to the appropriate authorities. Know what to report and to whom. Your report should include the name of the child care program. Be sure public health agencies are following up where there are implications of a child's illness for the rest of the children in the group.

Caring for Children With Chronic Conditions and Developmental/Behavioral Issues

When children have chronic medical conditions or developmental/behavioral problems, child care providers are often extensively involved in the care of the child. When you take the history of a chronic condition and when you make treatment recommendations, remember that the caregiver is a key partner in the care of the child. A multidisciplinary team approach can provide the optimal care for the child.

Obtaining Information From the Parents and Caregiver

Review the information on the child's signs and symptoms from parents and child care provider: When parents bring their child to you with concerns about the child's development or behavior, the concerns may have been identified in child care. The parents have valuable information to share about the child's behavior at home, in daily household activities, and with family members and friends. The child care provider has the opportunity to observe the child in comparison with many other children their age, over an extended period of time, and throughout a wide range of developmentally challenging activities (eg, negotiating with their peers over the rules of a game, putting together puzzles, and climbing on the playground equipment). In addition, many child care providers have training in early childhood development and work experience that helps them identify children with developmental and behavioral problems.

"We were very concerned about the development of a child in our center. We observed him for months, discussed our concerns with the parents, and suggested a full developmental assessment. The parents took the child to their doctor who did a brief assessment in the office and said, 'He's within normal. He'll grow out of it.' Unfortunately, the child didn't end up getting the assessment and intervention he needed until kindergarten and we lost an important opportunity to help the child earlier." (Child care director)

"Our center referred a child to his pediatrician because we were concerned about possible hearing problems. The parents said that the doctor took the concerns very seriously 'because day care sent him.' The child got evaluated promptly and got the hearing aid that he needed. Now he's doing very well." (Teacher)

To gather as much information as possible about the child, it can be invaluable to have the child care providers carefully observe and document their concerns about the child's development and behavior. The caregiver's initial complaint may be, "It's difficult having this child in my class," "This child throws off the whole group," or "Something's not quite right with this child." Instruct caregivers to document specific observations (eg, "During circle time every day this week, Tanya refused to sit in the circle and ran off to the block area."), rather than general statements (eg, "Tanya just can't handle circle time."), value judgments (eg, "Tanya is bad."), or diagnoses (eg, "Tanya has ADHD.").

Dr Bruce Gach of Livermore, CA, says, "When I refer a child for developmental assessment, it's very helpful when the caregiver has provided written information detailing her observations of the child's behavior and specific concerns—I staple the child care report onto the referral."

Ask the parents about contributing factors at home and child care: Children's behavior and symptoms of chronic conditions occur in response to many factors in the child's home and child care environment. Consider the factors that contribute to the child's behavior or illness at child care as well as at home. For example,

- When a child has asthma attacks in child care, ask about what exposures and activities appear to trigger the episodes.
- When there are concerns about a child's behavior at child care, ask about the characteristics of the child care setting (eg, how many caregivers, how many children, how much space), the activities the child engages in, the degree of structure in the program, how the caregiver instructs the children in appropriate behavior, the particular triggers for the behavior of concern, and the strategies the caregiver has used to manage the behavior.

Offer to speak with the child care provider: When a child has a chronic medical condition or developmental/behavioral problem, it is crucial that the pediatrician work in partnership with the parents and child care provider in all phases of care—gathering the information, making the assessment, developing the intervention plan, and following up on progress. Ask the parent for written consent for you to talk directly with the caregiver. If you have special hours or special procedures for taking calls from caregivers, give instructions to the parents to share with the caregiver. Remember that early childhood professionals have busy schedules too. Approach the contact as you would one with another colleague.

"Child care providers have significant training and experience in child development. If parents and pediatricians have any questions about the child's behavior or development, they should call us—you'll find that our input can be invaluable in assessing and caring for the child." (Child care director)

Consider doing an on-site observation at the child care program: A picture is worth a thousand words. Observing the child in his daily environment, engaged in activities, and interacting with other children and adults can provide a wealth of information about the child's development, far more than you can gather in a few minutes in your office.

Dr Jim Poole of Raleigh, NC, says, "These parents brought their child to my office saying that the child care program was concerned about his development and behavior. I ran the child through a quick assessment in the office and he looked fine to me. But the child care provider urged me to visit the program and observe the child there. I'm glad that I did because I saw that the child in fact had some problems that we needed to work on. I learned to always listen to the caregiver."

Ann Parker, MD, a developmental pediatrician in Berkeley, CA, conducts on-site observations of children in child care programs. She says, "It's invaluable for me to observe the child in his regular child care environment—his mood, how he plays, how he interacts with other children and adults. I get a clearer picture of the child's development, temperament, and how he relates to his world. It helps me talk with the child about his child care world. And it helps me tailor any intervention to what the teacher can do. Over time, by getting to know the local child care programs first-hand, I know which programs are better for children with special needs and different temperamental styles so I can give parents guidance on choosing the right child care program for their child."

Developing the Treatment Plan With the Parents and Caregiver

Develop a written care plan for the child: To ensure the best possible care for a child with special needs in child care, it is helpful for all the partners in the care of the child—the pediatrician, parents, child care provider, and other specialists—to work together to develop a treatment plan for the child. Comprehensive plans help caregivers care for children with special needs in routine and emergency situations. For example:

- When a child has suspected, potential, or known disabilities (eg, developmental, speech/hearing, visual, or motor disability), advocate for the child to get assessment and services through the local school district and participate in the Individualized Education Plan (IEP) or Individualized Family Service Plan (IFSP) process.

- When a child has a chronic medical condition, such as asthma or sickle cell anemia, work with the parents, caregivers, and any other specialists needed to develop an individualized treatment plans also known as an "Individualized Health Plan." This plan should detail the child's medical condition, measures to promote the child's health, triggers to avoid, medications and information on medication administration, accommodations in activities and diet, signs of an acute illness episode, and what to do and who to call in an emergency. (See Child Care Resources: Sample Individualized Health Plan.)

"My child had severe allergies and eczema as an infant. The pediatrician and child care center worked closely together to treat the condition and allow him to continue to attend the center. I'm so thankful that the doctor and child care really cared about what was best for my son's health and well-being, and mine too." (Parent)

"When Jamal had his first asthma attack at Head Start, we didn't know what was happening until one teacher noticed him hunched over in the corner of the playground having trouble breathing. By that point it was so bad that we had to call 911 and he was hospitalized for a week. After he recovered, we got together Jamal's parents and doctor to develop a health plan. It's really helped us a lot. Now we know how to avoid Jamal's asthma triggers, recognize the early signs of an attack, and give him his medicine before he gets really bad. He hasn't needed to be hospitalized again all year." (Teacher)

Simplify treatment recommendations and medications: If a child needs special health procedures or medications, try to prescribe them in a way that is most convenient to administer; and make sure that the child care program has the necessary supplies and equipment—and training—to use them.

Report specified conditions to the necessary authorities: State law requires you to report certain communicable diseases as well as suspected child abuse to the appropriate authority. Your report should include the name of the child care program. Know what to report and to whom.

Level One: Summary of Recommendations for Pediatric Involvement

- **Talk With Families About Child Care:** The earlier and the more frequently you address child care concerns, the better. National guidelines for health supervision recommend that child care topics be part of "anticipatory guidance" at all well-child visits.

- **Stay informed:** Read about child care. Talk with people about child care. Visit different types of child care programs.

- **Underscore the importance of quality child care:** Discuss with parents how consistent, warm, and responsive care for their young child lays an important foundation for the child's healthy development.

- **Provide information on finding child care:** Give parents guidance, written information, and referrals to help them find child care.

- **Document the child care program in the child's medical chart:** Devote a place on the history form or add a sticker to the chart with the name and telephone number of the child care program.

- **Complete the admission requirements:** Make sure the child's immunizations and health screenings are up-to-date. Ask the parents to bring the health forms required by the child care program.

- **Develop care plans for children with special needs:** If the child has special health or developmental needs, discuss with parents the importance of sharing information and working together with the caregiver to meet the child's needs.

- **Provide anticipatory guidance:** When the child is cared for both at home and in child care, all the anticipatory guidance should be directed both toward parents and caregivers; the home environment and the child care environment.

❉ **Promote a 3-way partnership among pediatrician, parents, and caregivers:** Remind parents that it is best for their child's health and development when you all work together. Explain that sometimes it is helpful for you to communicate directly with the caregiver, such as when there are concerns about their child's development or medications. Ask the parent for written consent for you to communicate directly with the caregiver, if needed. Use a letter, a phone call, e-mail, fax, or a visit—whatever works best.

❉ **Ask the parents about contributing factors at home** and **child care:** Children's behavior and symptoms of acute and chronic conditions occur in response to many factors in the child's home and child care environment.

❉ **Simplify treatment recommendations and medications:** If medication or procedures are needed, try to prescribe them in a manner that is convenient to administer.

❉ **Discuss when the child can return to child care:** Be understanding of parents' need to return to work or school. Discuss sick-child care options for children who are ill and emphasize the importance of having back-up caregivers.

❉ **Document the child's condition for the caregiver:** The clearer the communication among the pediatrician, parents, and caregivers, the better.

❉ **Offer to speak with the child care provider:** When a child has a chronic medical condition or developmental/behavioral problem, it is crucial that the pediatrician work in partnership with the parents and child care provider in all phases of care.

❉ **Consider doing an on-site observation at the child care program:** A picture is worth a thousand words.

References

1. Shore R. *Rethinking the Brain: New Insights into Early Development.* New York, NY: Families and Work Institute; 1997

2. Heilburn S, Culkin ML. *Cost, Quality and Child Outcomes in Child Care Centers.* Denver, CO: University of Colorado; 1995

3. Galinsky E. *The Study of Children in Family Child Care and Relative Care.* New York, NY: Families and Work Institute; 1994

4. Brown H. Who's watching our children? *Parenting.* June/July 1999:116–131

5. Green M, ed. *Bright Futures: Guidelines for Health Supervision of Infants, Children, and Adolescents.* Arlington, VA: National Center for Education in Maternal and Child Health; 1994

6. Young KT, Davis K, Schoen C, Parker S. Listening to parents. A national survey of parents with young children. *Arch Pediatr Adolesc Med.* 1998;152:255–262

7. American Academy of Pediatrics. Periodic survey of fellows #41. Pediatricians' experiences with child care health and safety. Available at: http://www.aap.org/research/ps41exs.htm. Accessed September 13, 2001

8. *A Woman's Guide to Breastfeeding.* Elk Grove Village, IL: American Academy of Pediatrics; 1998

9. American Academy of Pediatrics. *2000 Red Book: Report of the Committee on Infectious Diseases.* Pickering LK, ed. 25th ed. Elk Grove Village, IL: American Academy of Pediatrics; 2000

10. American Public Health Association, American Academy of Pediatrics. *Caring for Our Children: National Health and Safety Performance Standards: Guidelines for Out-of-Home Child Care Programs.* Washington, DC: American Public Health Association; 1992

11. American Academy of Pediatrics, Pennsylvania Chapter. *Preparing for Illness: A Joint Responsibility for Parents and Caregivers. Developed by Pennsylvania Chapter, American Academy of Pediatrics* [pamphlet]. 4th ed. Washington, DC: National Association for the Education of Young Children; 1999

Level Two

Providing Health Consultation to Child Care Programs

Health issues in child care can range from simple to complex. Early childhood programs can handle most minor and routine health matters on their own, such as caring for a child's scraped knee. However, when programs face more complex health concerns, such as caring for children with chronic medical conditions, they can benefit greatly from expert health consultation. Pediatricians, as well as nurses, mental health professionals, nutritionists, and other health experts, may provide consultation to child care programs for all health-related issues ranging from simple to complex.

Providing health consultation to child care programs requires a special interest and commitment on the part of the pediatrician. But you may find that being a health consultant to child care programs can advance your personal and professional goals by

* Providing preventive services in your community
* Promoting your patients' development and preventing illness and injury in child care
* Saving on capitated services for your patients with chronic conditions by improving their management in child care
* Increasing parents' satisfaction with your services
* Expanding community outreach and marketing for your practice

Establishing Relationships With Child Care Programs

Reaching Out to Those Who Care for Young Children

Pediatricians can begin to develop relationships with child care providers in many different ways. You may get a call from a local child care provider and simply respond to their request, or you may need to do a little outreach to market your services.

Many pediatricians begin a relationship with the child care program that their own children attend. If you are interested in enhancing services to your current patients, you may contact the child care programs that your patients attend. You might offer services to child care programs near your office so you can stop by for a visit at lunchtime. If you are new to practice or interested in expanding your practice, you might contact child care programs in the communities where you hope to develop your patient base. Or, you might offer your services to local child care programs that tend to have greater need for health consultation such as programs that serve low-income children and families (eg, Head Start and state-funded programs), infants, children with special needs, and mildly ill children. Remember that, since child care staff are generally paid low wages, many centers struggle with high turnover and a constant need for training. Many center directors cannot afford substitutes and spend a lot of time managing daily problems of the operation. Put yourself in their shoes as you consider what would be most helpful. Don't be disappointed if your offers to help are not immediately appreciated. As with doctor-patient relationships, it takes time to determine what is needed and to develop trust.

J. Deborah Ferholt, MD, has been providing health consultation to child care centers and family child care providers in New Haven, CT, since her residency. She helped developed one of the child care programs at Yale University. Currently, she has a private practice and is on faculty at Yale University School of Nursing where she co-teaches a course for nurse practitioner students on child care health consultation.

Defining the Health Consultant Relationship

The relationship between a health consultant and a child care program is different from the relationship between the physician and an individual patient or family. Although some of the children in the child care program may be your patients, others will have their own primary health care professional. Be sure to promote and not interfere with families' relationships with their child's medical home. The health consultant's "patient" or "client" is the entire child care program. The focus of consultation is on health issues that apply to the children, families, and staff as a group.

Examples of group health issues for which child care programs may request consultation include

- What infection control measures are necessary to prevent the spread of disease in the child care program?
- What are important safety features of playground equipment to prevent injuries to children?
- What snacks are nutritious and interesting for children?
- What toilet-training and discipline practices are developmentally appropriate?
- What measures should be taken to prevent back injuries among staff?
- How can the program support staff caring for children and families affected by substance abuse, mental illness, or family violence?
- How can staff receive state mandated health checks, needed immunizations, and training at low cost?

Although the child care health consultant's focus is on group health issues, you can also help the child care program meet the special health needs of individual children within the context of the child care program. For example,

- If a child does not have a primary health care professional, or lacks insurance, you can encourage the caregiver to talk with the family about the importance of a medical home and offer referrals to your own and other practices, the local public health department or community health center, and public sources of health insurance.
- If a child has a chronic medical condition, you can help facilitate communication among the child care staff, family, and the child's primary health care professional and specialists, and assist in developing health protocols and training to enable the child care staff meet the child's health needs in child care.

The health consultant should link the child care program with other resources in the community. When child care programs have other consultants, such as mental health professionals, pediatric nurse practitioners, or nutritionists, try to coordinate your services. You also may need to collaborate with the government agencies that oversee child care, such as the department of public health for communicable disease outbreaks, and children's protective services and child care licensing for suspected child abuse or neglect or other issues.

Recognize the inherent limits to the consultant's role. The child care program engages the consultant to make observations and provide information and recommendations. The consultant is an "outside expert" and has no authority within the program to make decisions and ensure that the program follows the recommendations. However, the program is more likely to implement the consultant's recommendations if the consultant is empathetic, understands the constraints of child care operation, and establishes good communication with the program director. Implementation requires effective program management, a consultation, and planning process that involves the staff and families that may be affected by the changes. Ultimately, the consultant's role is to help the child care program develop its own capacity to gather information, access resources, and solve its own problems. (For a sample job description, see Child Care Resources: Child Care Health Consultant Job Description.)

Communicating With Early Childhood Educators

Health consultation is most effective when it is provided in the context of a trusting and consistent relationship between the consultant and the child care program. All the partners in child care—child care providers, families, and consultants—must recognize and respect each other's unique knowledge, experience, and feelings. Effective communication is essential. It is important to listen carefully, ask questions, and clarify the issues involved. Sometimes communication can be challenging because you may have different office procedures and time constraints, use different terminology, and have different approaches to problem-solving.

In establishing the relationship between the health consultant and the child care program, it can be helpful to discuss what the spectrum of responsibility will be and establish some practical guidelines for contacts. For example,

- Who is the contact or responsible person at the child care program—the director, a designated health coordinator or advocate, or any staff person or parent?
- How do you want the program to contact you— by telephone, e-mail, fax, or letter?
- When do you prefer the program to contact you— on a spontaneous basis, only during specific office hours, or on a regularly scheduled basis?
- What is the most effective way for caregivers to present you with observations, questions, and concerns?

Consultants should always try to demonstrate an appreciation for the particular circumstances of the child care program, its challenges, and its strengths. Be sure to prioritize the health concerns and avoid overwhelming the program with too many recommendations at one time. Make recommendations that reinforce and build on the positive things already being done, that are cost-effective, and are easily implemented. Give clear and simple advice, outlined verbally and in writing, if possible.

When you have the opportunity to work with a child care program over an extended period of time, you can develop a quality improvement plan that proceeds at a reasonable pace from addressing the most critical to less critical health concerns. Long-term consulting relationships also allow the opportunity to follow-up and evaluate progress, to revise the action plan if needed, and to achieve steady quality improvement over time.

Providing Health Consultation Services

Pediatricians can offer a broad range of health consultation services to early childhood programs. First, respond to the questions or needs that programs have identified. You also may advise child care providers on health issues of which they might not have been previously aware, such as new health recommendations and regulations that affect child care practices (eg, infant sleep position and immunizations), emerging health issues (eg, antibiotic-resistant bacteria), and concerns you may have identified at site visits.

Health consultation to child care programs may involve many services.

Conducting a Needs Assessment

Health consultation should be tailored to the needs of the individual child care program. Child care programs have different characteristics, health needs, and resources. Conduct an initial, brief needs assessment with the child care program director—in person, by telephone, or in writing—to become familiar with the program's general characteristics and specific health needs and resources. The following questions may guide you to define the programs characteristics:

- How long has the program been in operation?
- How many children and of what ages attend the program?
- How are children grouped and how many children are in each group?

- What special health care needs do these children currently have?
- How many staff members are with the program? Do they have any special health care needs?
- What are the hours of operation?
- Is the program accredited through an organization?
- Are there any special features of the program, children, or families served (teen parents, ethnic background, and migrant workers)?
- What are the program's needs concerning health policies; staff, parent, or child training on health issues; and specific health issues noted from the last licensing visit?

The initial needs assessment process also can help the child care director get to know you, your areas of expertise, style of interaction, and availability. Together, you can identify what the child care program wants and needs, and determine whether that matches your expertise and availability. Some programs might need only a brief or limited consultation; other programs might want an ongoing relationship with a health consultant to address a broad range of health issues.

Visiting the Program—Observing Practices and Facilities

Visiting the child care site helps you understand the individual child care program and get to know the health concerns of the staff, parents, and children. The program may request a site visit for a particular concern, such as observing infection control practices associated with a disease outbreak, or for a comprehensive observation.

Take the time to observe the children and staff engaged in a full range of activities including drop-off, quiet and active play, food service, naptime, and diapering/toileting. Observe the quality of caregiver-child interactions and how well the child care program meets key standards for supervision, infection control, safety, nutrition, and developmentally appropriate practice. Inspect the entire facility, including entrances, exits, and hallways; indoor and outdoor play areas; food preparation areas; and child and adult bathrooms. Checklists can help organize the assessment but should be used with care to avoid intimidating child care providers and parents.[1]

After the site visit, meet with the program director to summarize the program's strengths, identify the most important health concerns, and discuss plans for improvement.

"When we had outbreaks of RSV and rotavirus that affected most of the infants in our center, I got worried and called our health consultant. She visited the center and did a thorough observation of our infection control practices. We sent a letter to parents about how we were addressing the problem, and everyone was greatly relieved." (Child care center director)

Karen Sokal-Gutierrez, MD, of Piedmont, CA, the health consultant for the above child care center, further describes the situation. "When the director called me about the RSV and rotavirus outbreaks, I asked, 'How have you handled it so far?' It sounded like they were doing all the right things. When I visited, I observed some excellent infection control practices and some problems. I couldn't have gotten the full picture over the phone—I had to see it with my own eyes. And meeting in person with staff helped to gather more information and be responsive to their needs and concerns."

Developing and Reviewing Child Care Health Policies

Every early childhood program needs written health policies that cover a broad range of child and staff health concerns. Child care health policies typically address discipline, safety, emergency preparedness, health screening, immunization, infection control, medications, and exclusion/readmission for illness. The health policies should be consistent with recommendations from the American Academy of Pediatrics and the American Public Health Association, federal regulations such as the Americans with Disabilities Act (ADA) and Occupational Safety and Health Administration (OSHA) Blood-borne Pathogens Regulations, and state licensing regulations and medical/nurse practice acts.

You can use a model health policy to help programs develop new health policies or revise existing health policies.[1]

"Our preschool hadn't updated its health policies in many years. So I asked our health consultant to review them. Our illness exclusion policy had become a source of conflict with parents—they felt we were sending children home too much. Our consultant told us that we didn't need to exclude children for runny noses, low-grade fevers, and hand-foot-and-mouth syndrome. Our parents are a lot happier and we are more confident of our policy." (Preschool director)

Ensuring Medical Homes and Preventive Care

Help the child care program ensure that all of the children have a medical home and receive well-child care, screening, diagnosis, and treatment for any special health needs. When children lack a medical home, you can provide referrals to your practice and other primary health care professionals in the community. In some cases, you might provide on-site child health screenings such as physical examinations, developmental screenings, and vision and hearing tests. Always send the results of these services to an ongoing source of health care for the child. You also can help the program interpret the results of children's health assessments and the implications for their care. For more information about medical homes for children, the AAP Web site offers electronic versions of the policy statements, "The Medical Home"[2] and "The Medical Home Statement Addendum: Pediatric Primary Health Care."[3] (See Child Care Resources.)

Developing Plans to Care for Children With Chronic Conditions

Help ensure that child care staff is prepared to care for children with special needs in the program. Work with the child care staff, family, and their health care professionals to gather the necessary information and develop a plan for the child's routine and emergency care in the program. Health forms that detail accommodations in activities, nutrition, medications, health procedures, equipment, and facilities are useful. (See Child Care Resources: Sample Individualized Health Plan.) Help the program make sure that medications and supplies are on hand, staff is trained in necessary procedures, and emergency medical back-up is available. Work with the child care provider, family, and the child's health care professionals to periodically review and revise the special care plans. Assist child care providers to work with specialists as necessary to ensure medication administration and procedures are performed appropriately.

"For the past 3 years, our center has cared for a child with diabetes. The child's parents and pediatrician have provided us with most of the information we need to care for the child. But our health consultant has really helped address staff concerns and problem solve when difficulties have arisen. She doesn't just give us the medical information but she helps us apply it to child care." (Child care director)

Providing Health Education for Staff, Parents, and Children

Work with the program director to identify the program's health training needs. The training topics may be based on state licensing requirements, specific health concerns that the program has experienced, problem areas identified at your site visit or their licensing visit, or new "hot topics" in child health. (See Level Three: Conducting Workshops on Child Development, Health, and Safety.)

You might provide the training or help identify other health specialists who can provide the training. Separate or joint workshops can be conducted for staff and parents. You also might offer health education for the children on topics such as hand washing, toothbrushing, eating healthy foods, and medical/dental check ups. Health education for staff, parents, and children is most effective when it builds on the experiences of participants, uses audiovisual aids, and allows for active participation.

"Our health consultant provides yearly in-service training on health issues for our staff. He has a great way of making the technical information clear and simple to understand. He also appreciates what we do in child care and understands the parents' perspective, which is very important." (Child care provider)

A group of more than 20 physicians and nurse practitioners at Boston Medical Center organized a project, Healthy Child Care Boston, that provides health consultation to family child care homes in the city. They do "house call" visits to family child care homes for question-and-answer sessions on child development, health, and safety.

Reviewing Illness and Injury Logs

Advise child care programs to keep records of illnesses and injuries that children and staff experience in their program. The form should describe the illness or injury and what action was taken. (See Child Care Resources: Symptom Record and Injury Report Form.) This documentation can be helpful for health care follow up and for legal review, if necessary.

Help the program review the illness and injury logs periodically to identify patterns of concern, such as outbreaks of certain kinds of diseases or equipment frequently involved in injuries. Based on the patterns of illnesses and injuries noted, work with the staff to

develop plans to improve the prevention and management of illness and injury in the program.

"Our child care program's health consultant helped us review our records of children's and staff injuries. We found that one piece of play equipment caused too many injuries, so we removed it. We also had a problem with staff back injuries. So our consultant did a workshop for staff on back safety. We reviewed the basic principles of bending and lifting and we developed specific strategies to protect our backs in each of our activities caring for children. It was very helpful." (Child care teacher)

Providing Ongoing Health Consultation

Child care programs can benefit from having an ongoing relationship with a pediatrician consultant who is available to address whatever health issues may arise. For example, a child care program might call you to ask how it can stop the head lice outbreak that has been occurring in the center for a month. If you have visited the center and are familiar with the routines and facilities, such as the popularity of "dress-up" play and the arrangement of children's clothes in the cubbies, your recommendations can address that particular situation. You can provide information and advice over the telephone or on site, and/or refer the program to resources such as written or video materials. For sensitive issues, such as working with the families whose children have chronic head lice infestations, a trusting relationship between the health consultant, child care providers, and families can be invaluable. The health consultant can help clarify the issues and facilitate communication among the child care providers, parents, and other service providers, when necessary. The roles and responsibilities of a child care health consultant are elaborated in the attached child care health consultant job description. (See Child Care Resources: Child Care Health Consultant Job Description.)

"When we started with our health consultant years ago, we used to call with questions about the common infectious diseases. But over time, she's taught us a lot about the common illnesses and given us resources to manage them on our own. Now we mostly call for the difficult questions, like caring for children with chronic medical conditions." (Child care director)

"When I got a call from a parent inquiring about enrolling her child who had a rare degenerative neurological disorder, I was a bit overwhelmed. I almost didn't know where to begin to think about how to care for the child. Our health consultant helped us think through the questions systematically: What were the child's care needs now? What was anticipated in the future? What accommodations would the center need to make to care for the child? Was this the best setting for the child? The health consultant helped us see that, whatever the medical condition, there was a process we could go through to determine whether we could care for a child." (Child care director)

Legal Issues for Health Consultants

Laws and Regulations

Consultants who provide health consultation services to child care programs must know the laws and regulations that apply. These include child care licensing regulations, health and safety codes, medical/nurse practice acts; Early Intervention and Special Education laws; the ADA, OSHA regulations, and Head Start Program Performance Standards. Also, consultants should know the child care program requirements for health consultation (eg, some states require monthly health visits to infant centers), and the health training requirements for child care providers (eg, some states require training in first aid and infection control).

The consultant should be familiar with state requirements for reporting incidents occurring in child care, such as suspected child abuse and neglect and certain communicable diseases. The consultant should know what is reportable and how and to whom to make reports. Additional information about OSHA regulations for pediatric practices can be obtained by contacting the Health Policy Analyst in the AAP Division of Health Care Finance and Practice at 800/433-9016. (For more information about child care health and safety regulations and laws, see Child Care References.)

Consent and Confidentiality

If the child care program has requested for the provision of direct services for individual children, such as health screening, the consent of the child's parent or legal guardian is required. If necessary, parental consent is required to contact a child's health care professional. Medical information about a child should be discussed only with individuals who need to know to care for the child, and then only with the written consent of the parents or legal guardian.

Liability

To provide the highest standard of care and to limit the liability for consulting activities, use the most current recommendations from national authorities such as the AAP, the APHA, and the Centers for Disease Control and Prevention (CDC). (See Child Care Resources.) You can take continuing medical education courses and subscribe to relevant child care health and safety publications, or access the Web sites where this material is kept up-to-date. (See Child Care Resources.) In addition, keep a health record that includes a written record of the date, the client, the reason for consultation, and the information or advice provided for each health consultation. Consultants should share a description of the child care responsibilities with their medical malpractice insurance carrier and ask for written confirmation of coverage for these activities, noting any restrictions and/or the need to add additional coverage. For additional information, contact the Health Policy Analyst in the AAP Division of Health Care Finance and Practice at 800/433-9016.

Financial Issues for Health Consultants

Pediatricians who provide health consultation to child care programs may choose to donate or charge for their services.

Volunteer Services

Most child care programs have limited funds and appreciate receiving free consulting services. Consultants should consider providing free child care health consultation as part of their overall service to the community. Also, consultants could provide free services to a certain number of hours per year, or offer free services to programs serving low-income children and families.

Paid Services

Some child care programs have financial resources to pay for health consultation and training. When a consultant is paid for services, then expectations and accountability is clear. Health consultants may charge child care programs a fee for specific services or for consultation time. Consultants may have a fixed rate or a sliding scale depending on the needs and resources of the child care program. Also, consultants may be able to bill health insurance companies or Medicaid for direct medical services provided at the child care facility as they would at the office or clinic. Governmental agencies (eg, the US

Department of Health and Human Services and the Department of Education), foundations, service organizations, and corporations also may provide grants for health consultation or research projects with child care programs. In addition, pediatricians might consider working with the AAP Department of Community Pediatrics to develop a Community Access To Child Health Program (CATCH). For more information, contact the CATCH program at 800/433-9016, ext 7632.

Level Two: Summary of Recommendations for Pediatric Involvement

1. *Build relationships with child care providers.* Begin a relationship with the child care programs that your patients attend. Offer your services to local child care programs that tend to have greater need for health consultation such as programs that serve low-income children and families, infants, children with special needs, and mildly ill children.

2. *Ensure that each child has a medical home.* Encourage caregivers to talk with families about the importance of a medical home and offer referrals to your own and other practices, the local public health department, or community health clinic.

3. *Promote effective communication.* Develop a trusting and consistent relationship with the child care program by recognizing and respecting each other's unique knowledge, experience, and feelings.

4. *Assess the child care program health needs.* Health consultation should be tailored to the needs of the individual child care program. Child care programs have different characteristics, health needs, and resources. Conduct an initial, brief needs assessment with the child care program director—in person, by telephone, or in writing.

5. *Develop and review child care health policies.* Every early childhood program needs written health policies that cover a broad range of child and staff health concerns. Child care health policies typically address discipline, safety, emergency preparedness, health screening, immunization, infection control, medications, and exclusion/readmission for illness.

6. *Develop plans for caring for children with chronic conditions.* Help ensure that the child care staff is prepared to care for children with special health care needs in the program. Help develop written care plans and ensure that staff is knowledgeable about special education programs and trained to administer needed medications, procedures, and emergency plans.

7. *Conduct health education for staff, parents, and children.* You can provide or help arrange training on a wide range of health and safety topics. Health education for staff, parents, and children is most effective when it builds on the experiences of participants, uses audiovisual aids, and allows for active participation.

8. *Liability.* To provide the highest standard of care and to limit your liability for consulting activities, follow the most current recommendations from national authorities such as the AAP, the APHA, and the CDC. Be sure to get a letter from your carrier that includes coverage for the work you plan to do.

References

1. Aronson S, Smith H, eds. *Model Child Care Health Policies.* Bryn Mawr, PA: Pennsylvania Chapter of the American Academy of Pediatrics; 1997

2. American Academy of Pediatrics, Ad Hoc Task Force on Definition of the Medical Home. The medical home. *Pediatrics.* 1992;90:774

3. American Academy of Pediatrics. The medical home statement addendum: pediatric primary health care. *AAP News.* November 1993:7

Level Three

Advocating for Quality Child Care

After informing yourself about child care, helping your patients find the best child care for their child, and working directly with one or more child care providers in your community, you might want to work on improving the quality of child care available in your community. For example,

⁜ You might discover that it is difficult to find a local preschool that meets the needs of your patients with developmental delay. You think that the preschools might benefit from better training and support on caring for children with special needs.

⁜ You might find that several of your patients who attend the same child care program have suffered recurrent bouts of diarrhea illness. You think that the center staff might benefit from better training and monitoring on infection control.

⁜ You might hear about the high rate of turnover of caregivers (generally 30% to 40% per year) and be concerned about its impact on early childhood relationships and development. You think that better financing and support for caregivers might help promote stable caregiving relationships and early childhood development.

You can take the important next step—advocating for improvements in the quality of child care in your community.

Providing Assistance to a Local Child Care Program

Consider working with a local child care program to improve child health. You can help by doing the following:

Serving on an Advisory Board

Offer to serve on a child care advisory board such as the health advisory committee for a local Head Start program or the Board of Directors of a local program or the child care resource and referral agency. By doing so, you can help ensure that the children have medical homes, caregivers receive adequate training in health and safety, and the child care facilities are safe.

Tom Tonniges, MD, said, "When I set up practice in Nebraska, I visited the local Head Start center and participated on the Board of another center. Pretty soon, word got around to families that we were the pediatricians who cared about children in the community. It was good for children and families, and great marketing for our practice."

Conducting Workshops on Child Development, Health, and Safety

You can offer health education workshops for child care staff and parents. The training topics may be based on state licensing requirements, specific health concerns that the program has experienced, or new "hot topics" in child health. Common topics for health training include the following:

⁜ Child Growth and Development
⁜ Promoting Breastfeeding
⁜ Promoting Mental Health
⁜ Managing Challenging Behavior
⁜ Inclusive Child Care
⁜ Common Childhood Illnesses
⁜ Communicable Disease Prevention and Management
⁜ Injury Prevention and Emergency Preparedness
⁜ First Aid
⁜ Playground Safety
⁜ Nutrition and Food Safety
⁜ Caring for Children With Chronic Conditions
⁜ Child Abuse Prevention and Response
⁜ Child Passenger Safety
⁜ Staff Health Issues
⁜ Communicating With Parents About Health and Safety
⁜ Using Pediatricians as a Resource on Health and Safety

You also can help plan health education for the children on topics such as hand washing, toothbrushing, eating healthy foods, and the importance of regular medical/dental check ups. Health education for staff, parents, and children is most effective when it builds on the experiences of participants, uses audiovisual aids, and allows for active participation. For a copy of a sample curriculum on one of the above topics, contact the corresponding organization listed in the reference section of this manual.

"Our preschool has had some parents who are pediatricians. They've been very helpful in doing parent education on different child development and health issues. They've also done circle time for the children about their job as doctors and why it's important for the children to get shots. One pediatrician put together doctor's kits for children's dramatic play. It's been very enriching for our program." (Teacher)

Donating or Advocating for Additional Services, Supplies, or Funding

Consider donating supplies, money, or your services as a health consultant to a local child care program (see Level Two: Providing Health Consultation to Child Care Programs). Donations of supplies and money to a non-profit program are usually tax deductible. Supplies that might be helpful for a child care program include the following:

※ Computers, office equipment, and supplies

※ Medical supplies (eg, latex gloves, disinfectant, peak flow meter, nebulizer)

※ Educational materials on child development, health, and safety (eg, books, videos, CD-ROMs, and brochures). Some of the AAP parent education brochures that are particularly helpful for child care programs are

> ❖ What Parents Need to Know About Vaccines and Childhood Diseases
> ❖ Your Child's Eyes
> ❖ A Guide to Children's Dental Health
> ❖ Choking Prevention and First Aid for Infants and Children
> ❖ Protect Your Child From Poison
> ❖ Fun in the Sun: Keep Your Baby Safe
> ❖ Toilet Training
> ❖ Better Health and Fitness Through Physical Activity
> ❖ Playground Safety
> ❖ Common Childhood Infections
> ❖ Ear Infections and Children
> ❖ Allergies in Children
> ❖ Learning Disabilities and Children
> ❖ Understanding the Child With ADHD

"In the pediatrician's office I just saw the AAP brochures for parent education. There are so many that would be fantastic for our child care program. I wish we could have the entire set available at our program—it'd be helpful for staff and parents." (Child care director)

Promoting Early Childhood Professional Development

Reach out to child care professionals and provide information on child health and safety. You can start by doing the following:

Participating in Early Childhood Professional Organizations and Conferences

Join a local early childhood organization such as the local chapter of the National Association for the Education of Young Children (NAEYC). Contact the coordinators of early childhood conferences to offer workshops or question-and-answer sessions on child development, health, and safety. Conferences may be sponsored by the local child care resource and referral agency, child care regulatory or subsidy agency, local chapter of the NAEYC, or a family child care association. Community college and university early childhood education courses might also welcome a guest speaker on child development, health, and safety.

The AAP Committee on Early Childhood, Adoption, and Dependent Care sponsors a half-day session at the annual NAEYC conference. Committee members and other pediatricians present information on important topics in child health, and then address participants' questions about a wide range of child development, health, and safety issues. An early childhood professional said, "I find the annual AAP session very helpful. I wish we could do the same with local pediatricians at our local AEYC conference."

Writing Articles on Health for Child Care Publications

Contact the publishers of child care publications and offer to write articles on health. Local child care associations, child care resource and referral agencies, and university extension offices may have newsletters for child care providers.

Susan Aronson, MD, a pediatrician in Philadelphia, writes a column for the nationally distributed Child Care Information Exchange magazine; and Phil Chamberlain, MD, of Oakland, CA, writes a column on children's health for the local Parents' Press. A child care provider said, "I always look forward to reading the articles on health. Even with my years of experience, I always learn something new that I can apply in my work with children and families."

Providing Consultation to Agencies That Offer Child Care Technical Assistance

Develop a relationship with local agencies that provide technical assistance to child care professionals: the child care resource and referral agency, child care licensing agency, and family child care associations. Help update them about new health recommendations, such as immunizations or infant sleep position, so they can disseminate current health information to child care providers.

> **For a listing of the child care resource and referral agency nearest you, contact the National Child Care Aware Organization at 800/424-2246.**

Dr Aronson and the AAP Pennsylvania Chapter work closely with the state child care licensing agency. The AAP Pennsylvania Chapter has helped the licensing agency update the regulations to conform with the health and safety standards recommended in Caring for Our Children. *It also has provided written guidance, technical assistance, and training to licensing administrators to assist them as they look for health and safety features during child care site visits, as well as ways that they can help child care programs meet the national health and safety standards. It brings AAP information to the attention of the regulators, child care resource and referral agencies, and the organizations for child care providers in the state who, in turn, help make sure caregivers and parents are kept informed.*

Advocating for Improved Supply, Financing, and Regulation of Child Care

Every state in the country is currently conducting a review of the supply and quality of child care to meet the need for child care with welfare reform and other demographic changes. Pediatricians can play a key role advocating for improving the supply, financing, and quality of child care to promote child development, health, and safety. You can help by doing the following:

Serving on Child Care Planning Committees

Help keep children's health and safety on the political agenda and ensure that the plans for child care promote children's development, health, and safety. Join your state AAP Committee on Early Childhood, Adoption, and Dependent Care. Participate on local or statewide Advisory Committees overseeing child care planning, policies, funding, and regulation. Join other child advocacy groups to sponsor legislation and regulations promoting quality child care and provide oral and written comments on proposed legislation and regulations.

Estelle Siker, MD, was employed at the Connecticut Department of Public Health for many years and was instrumental in strengthening the state child care regulations. Collaborating with nursing, early childhood, and public health professionals, Dr Siker advocated for regulations requiring health, dental, social service, and nutritional consultation to child care programs. She is currently the co-chair of the Connecticut AAP Chapter Committee on Early Childhood, Adoption, and Dependent Care.

Peter Michael Miller, MD, Howard Taras, MD, Jogi Khanna, MD, Bruce Gach, MD, Birt Harvey, MD, Robert Ross, MD, Robert Byrd, MD, and other members of the California AAP Chapter participated in statewide planning forums coordinated by the California Healthy Child Care campaign. Pediatricians worked with representatives of the state Departments of Health, Education, and Social Services, and other groups to develop plans to upgrade health and safety regulations in child care, ensure medical homes and well-child care, facilitate the care of children with special needs in child care, standardize health and safety training for caregivers, and promote health consultation to child care programs.

Working With Child Care and Child Health Advocacy Organizations

Start close to home. If you work in a hospital or office park, is there a need for on-site child care? Survey other workers and advocate for high-quality, on-site child care, if needed.

Bright Horizons Family Solutions operates on-site child care centers at many hospitals and office parks across the country. A parent who is a physician said, "I feel confident that my children receive the highest quality care at the center. It helped me feel comfortable going back to work knowing that I could visit to breastfeed my infant and have lunch with my preschooler. When I'm comfortable with the child care, I feel more satisfied with my work."

Advocate on local, statewide, and national levels to promote breastfeeding, mental health services, inclusion for children with special needs, and child health insurance. Join with early childhood professional groups that advocate for improving the supply and quality of child care and securing adequate wages and benefits for child care workers. Contact the Center for Child Care Workforce and other early childhood organizations that sponsor the "Worthy Wage Campaign." (See Child Care Resources.)

Review the AAP policy statement, *The Pediatrician's Role in Community Pediatrics,*[1] to reexamine and reaffirm your role as a community pediatrician, examine a concise definition of community pediatrics, and review AAP recommendations that underscore the critical nature of this important dimension of your profession.

Contacting Local Media to Gain Interest in and Exposure for Promoting Quality Child Care

Working with the media is an effective way to reach partners in your community with important information about healthy and safe child care environments. Establish your reputation as an expert in child health with ready access to relevant data. Remember that personal stories are the essential ingredient in a good news story. Use the following ideas to generate interest:

❖ Emphasize the importance that quality child care plays in a child's development.

❖ Talk about how nutrition, injury and infectious disease prevention, and developmentally appropriate educational activities (all components of high-quality child care programs) contribute to a child's healthy development.

❖ Discuss the high turnover rate of those who care for young children and describe ways parents and child care and health professionals can work together to improve this situation.

❖ Encourage local child care provider attendance at educational sessions that you plan to present and explain how educating child care professionals can be instrumental in detecting possible areas of concern and referring children to their medical home for follow-up.

Legislative Advocacy

Successfully advocating for children can be an incredibly rewarding experience. Legislators can be effective partners in promoting child health and making things happen when other attempts have failed. You can become an effective advocate for children by: (1) developing credibility in the community through community service and networking, (2) understanding the legislative process by becoming involved in attempting to pass legislation, and (3) working proactively as a recognized expert in a child health policy by appropriate policy makers. More information is available in a commentary entitled "Training Pediatricians to Become Child Advocates," by Steve Berman, MD, FAAP, published in the September 1998 issue of *Pediatrics.*[2]

Developing a Health and Safety Initiative in Child Care

Pediatricians and early childhood professionals have a common interest in promoting child development, health, and safety. Join local child care professionals to develop a community-based child/health initiative. Consider the following:

Conducting Research on Health and Safety in Child Care

With the dramatic increase in the numbers of children in child care in recent years, there is a growing need for research on children's development, health, and safety in child care. Collaborate with early childhood programs to collect data or conduct research on health-related issues.

Al Chang, MD, at San Diego State University School of Public Health, directed a project funded by the Centers for Disease Control to study the rates and causes of injuries in child care programs.

Jody Murph, MD, an infectious disease specialist at Children's Hospital of Iowa, directs a research project funded by National Institute for Child Health and Development on infectious diseases in child care. The project has hired and trained nurse health consultants to work with child care programs with the aim of reducing infectious diseases among children and staff in child care.

Sponsoring a Community-Based Health Promotion Project

Work with child care providers in your community to build on child health promotion initiatives sponsored by the AAP, the Maternal and Child Health Bureau (MCHB), and other national organizations. For example,

❊ Join your state Healthy Child Care America Project. Serve on statewide or local planning committees and offer to provide services that may be needed in your area such as advocacy for child care legislation, health workshops, consultation to child care programs, or a medical home for children.

❊ Use the AAP Speaker's Kit on Breastfeeding Promotion and Management (see Child Care Resources). Work with local child care organizations to develop child care policies and facilities to promote breastfeeding, display posters, and provide workshops for parents and staff on the benefits of breastfeeding. Set up an evaluation to document changes in breastfeeding practices.

❊ Use the Moving Kids Safely in Child Care: A Child Passenger Safety Resource Kit for Child Care Providers (see Child Care Resources). Work with local child care organizations to develop safe transportation policies for child care programs and provide education for parents and staff on the proper use of car seats, seat belts, and air bags.

❊ Use the AAP *Preparing for Illness* brochure. (See Child Care Resources.) Help local child care providers develop appropriate policies for inclusion and exclusion of children from care. For model child care health policies, encourage child care providers to adapt the AAP *Model Child Care Health Policies* to plan for a safe and healthy program.

Increasing the Involvement of Health Professionals in Child Care

Talk about child care with your health professional colleagues—physicians, dentists, nurses, mental health professionals, health educators, etc. Encourage your colleagues to get involved in child care.

Teaching Pediatric Residents About Child Care

If you are on the faculty of a university, medical school, or hospital residency program, incorporate child care health and safety issues into your curriculum.

Lewis First, MD, Director of Pediatrics at the University of Vermont, teaches pediatric residents about children's health in child care. Pediatric residents visit child care programs for their rotation on Child Development and serve as health consultants for child care programs as part of their continuity clinic, over the course of their residency.

Neal Kaufman, MD, at the Cedars-Sinai Medical Center in Los Angeles, developed a comprehensive course for pediatric residents on child development, health, and safety in child care. The curriculum involves readings, observations at child care programs, and practice providing training and health consultation to child care providers.

Participating in Continuing Medical Education on Child Care

Participate in continuing education activities on child development, health, and safety in child care. These may include grand rounds at your local hospital or statewide and national pediatric conferences.

The North Carolina Pediatric Society collaborated with the University of North Carolina at Chapel Hill and the North Carolina Department of Health to develop a 1-hour slide presentation and script for pediatric grand rounds on health and safety in child care. The grand rounds presentation has helped increase pediatricians' awareness of health issues in child care.

Pediatricians in several states are collaborating with the Healthy Child Care America project funded by the Maternal and Child Health Bureau. Ed Schor, MD, at the Iowa Department of Health directs the Healthy Child Care Iowa project that has recruited and trained public health nurses across the state to provide health consultation to local child care programs. Judith Romano, MD, works with the West Virginia Chapter of AAP and the Healthy Child Care West Virginia project, which is also recruiting pediatricians and other health professionals to serve as health consultants to child care programs.

Level Three: Summary of Recommendations for Pediatric Involvement

※ *Serve on the advisory board:* Offer to serve on a child care advisory board such as the health advisory committee for a local Head Start program or the Board of Directors of the child care resource and referral agency.

※ *Conduct workshops on child development, health, and safety:* Offer health workshops for child care staff, parents, and children.

※ *Participate in early childhood professional organizations and conferences:* Join a local early childhood organization. Contact the coordinators of early childhood conferences to offer workshops or question-and-answer sessions on child development, health, and safety.

※ *Contact the publishers of child care publications and offer to write articles on health:* Local child care associations, child care resource and referral agencies, and university extension offices may have newsletters for child care providers.

※ *Develop a relationship with local agencies that provide technical assistance to child care professionals:* The child care resource and referral agency, child care licensing agency, and family child care associations typically provide this type of assistance.

※ *Serve on a child care planning committee:* Help keep children's health and safety on the political agenda and ensure that the plans for child care promote children's development, health, and safety.

※ *Conduct research on health and safety in child care:* Collaborate with early childhood programs to conduct research.

※ *Teach pediatric residents about child care:* If you are on the faculty of a university, medical school, or hospital residency program, incorporate child care health and safety issues into your curriculum.

※ *Participate in continuing education on child care:* This may include grand rounds at your local hospital or statewide and national pediatric conferences.

References

1. American Academy of Pediatrics, Committee on Community Health Services. The pediatrician's role in community pediatrics. *Pediatrics*. 1999;103:1304–1306

2. Berman S. Training pediatricians to become child advocates [commentary]. *Pediatrics*. 1998;102:632–635

Summary

Promoting Health and Safety in Child Care: Different Levels of Involvement for Pediatricians

❈ ❈ ❈ ❈ ❈ ❈ ❈ ❈ ❈ ❈ ❈ ❈ ❈ ❈

Summary

The quality of child care that children receive in their early years is crucial for their development, health, and safety. You can help promote health and safety in child care through encouraging a 3-way partnership among pediatricians, parents, and child care providers. By talking with parents about child care, working with child care programs, and advocating for quality child care, you can make a significant contribution to the health and well-being of children and families.

Increase your involvement in child care programs and local health and safety initiatives.

Integrate child care issues throughout all aspects of your pediatric practice. At well-child visits, beginning with the prenatal visit, ask families about their child care plans and listen to their experiences and concerns. Refer families to local child care resource and referral services. Talk with families about the different types of child care, how to identify quality care, and how to assess whether the child care meets their child's and family's needs. Offer families tips on preparing for the transition to child care, and be sure to follow up and support them in their child care decisions. In caring for children with acute or chronic conditions, remember to work with both the family and the caregivers to thoroughly assess the child's condition and develop workable treatment plans.

Reach out to provide health consultation to local child care programs. Talk with child care directors, staff, and families to help them assess their health needs. Visit child care programs to observe the facilities and health and safety practices. Assist child care programs in reviewing health policies, ensuring medical homes for children, and developing plans for the care of children with chronic conditions. Offer health education for staff, parents, and children. In addition, be available on an ongoing basis to address health concerns that may arise.

Advocate for quality child care in your community. Offer to serve on a child care advisory board or planning committee. Provide expert testimony to support local, state, or national child care initiatives. Contribute to early childhood professional development by writing articles or offering workshops on health and safety. Consider encouraging the collection of data or conducting research as well as teaching pediatric residents and other health professionals about health and safety in child care.

Remember, by working as partners with parents and caregivers, you can make a difference in the lives of children and families.

General
Child Care
Information

General Child Care Information

The following components are included to assist you as you begin your activities in child care. This information is useful for all 3 levels of pediatrician involvement.

⁂ Key Facts on Child Care and Early Education
⁂ The Importance of Quality Child Care
⁂ Types of Child Care
⁂ Helping Parents Transition Their Child Into Child Care
⁂ Special Health Considerations for Child Care
⁂ Infectious Diseases in Child Care Programs
⁂ Planning for the Care of Ill Children
⁂ Child Care for Children With Special Needs

Key Facts on Child Care and Early Education

Percentages of children in child care:

⁂ By the age of 6, 84% of children have received supplemental child care and education.[1]
⁂ Percentage of mothers in the workforce when their youngest child is…[1]
  ❖ Under age 1: 57%
  ❖ Under age 3: 59%
  ❖ Under age 6: 62%
  ❖ 6–13 years: 75%

The types of child care families use include:[2]

⁂ Parents: 22%
⁂ Relatives, in the child's or relative's home: 25%
⁂ Nonrelative, in the child's home: 5%
⁂ Nonrelative, in the caregiver's home: 17%
⁂ Child care facilities (centers, nursery schools, preschools): 30%

Concerns about child care:

⁂ A study of child care centers in the United States found that only 14% of centers had high-quality care, 74% provided mediocre care, and 12% threatened the health and safety of children. Infant/toddler care was of greatest concern with only 8% providing high-quality care and 40% endangering children's health and safety.[3]

⁂ A study of family child care homes found that only 9% provided high-quality care, 56% provided barely adequate care, and 35% provided poor-quality care.[4]
⁂ The turnover rate for child care center providers is 36% per year.[3]
⁂ Children in child care, especially infants, are at increased risk for infectious diseases such as ear infections, pneumonia, and diarrheal illness.[5]

The Importance of Quality Child Care

⁂ Children who attend high-quality child care have cognitive and socio-emotional advantages that persist through the early school years. Children who attended child care with higher quality classroom practices were found to have better language and math skills, and children who had closer relationships with their child care teachers were found to have better classroom behavior and social skills. Children whose mothers had lower levels of education— who are at greater risk for school difficulties— experienced the greatest benefits from high-quality child care.[6]
⁂ Higher quality child care for very young children (birth to 3 years) was consistently related to high levels of cognitive and language development.[7]
⁂ Children who receive warm and sensitive caregiving are more likely to trust caregivers, to enter school ready and eager to learn, and to get along well with other children.[8]
⁂ Smaller group sizes, higher teacher-child ratios, and higher staff wages are associated with quality child care.[3]
⁂ States with stronger licensing requirements had a greater number of good-quality centers.[3]
⁂ Voluntary conformity to higher standards through professional center accreditation or through meeting another set of quality standards also increased the likelihood of higher classroom quality.[3]

Types of Child Care*

❉ ❉ ❉ ❉ ❉ ❉

Type of Care	Advantages	Disadvantages
In-Home Care: The caregiver cares for the child in the child's home.	❊ The child stays in familiar surroundings. ❊ The child receives individualized care and attention. ❊ Limited exposure to infectious diseases. ❊ The caregiver may do light housework as well as child care. ❊ Less transportation involved.	❊ Higher cost. Caregiver must make minimum wage, pay Social Security, and report taxes. ❊ May affect family privacy. ❊ Caregiver may have limited training in child development, health, and safety. ❊ May not have developmentally appropriate activities. ❊ Caregiver may have feelings of isolation. ❊ If caregiver gets sick, takes vacation, has a family crisis, or is suddenly unavailable, it may be difficult to find a replacement.
Family Child Care: The caregiver cares for the child in the caregiver's home. The caregiver also may care for children from his or her own family and other families.	❊ Less expensive than in-home care. ❊ Usually a small number of children and favorable adult-child ratio. ❊ Opportunity to play with other children. ❊ Comfort of a home setting. ❊ May be flexible to meet individual needs.	❊ Limited social support and supervision of caregiver. ❊ May have limited training in child development, health, and safety. ❊ May not have developmentally appropriate activities. ❊ If caregiver gets sick, takes vacation, has a family crisis, or is suddenly unavailable, it may be difficult to find a replacement. ❊ May be less likely to comply with state child care standards and policies.
Child care center or preschool: Caregivers or teachers care for the child within a group of children in a facility designed for young children.	❊ More likely to be regulated. ❊ Caregivers tend to be better trained and supervised. ❊ More likely to have a structured program designed to meet children's developmental needs. ❊ If a caregiver gets sick, takes vacation, has a family crisis, or is suddenly unavailable, a substitute is usually available. ❊ Includes additional monitoring, support, and education for the provider.	❊ May be more expensive than family child care. ❊ There may be a waiting list for admission. ❊ Child may be cared for in a larger group with less individualized attention and supervision. ❊ Child exposed to more infectious diseases.

*Adapted from American Academy of Pediatrics.[9]

Helping Parents Transition Their Child Into Child Care
❋ ❋ ❋ ❋ ❋ ❋

Child's Developmental Stage	Parents' Response
Birth to 7 months: In early infancy, babies primarily need love, comforting, and good basic care to satisfy their physical needs.	Though this period may be a difficult time of separation for parents, young infants generally will accommodate well to a consistent and nurturing caregiver in almost any setting. After the initial transition period, parents can stay for up to 1 hour. This can be shortened by the end of 1 to 2 weeks.
7 to 12 months: This is when stranger anxiety normally occurs. Babies may suddenly be reluctant to stay with anyone outside the family. The unfamiliar setting of child care may also upset them.	If possible, parents should try not to start child care during times when a child is experiencing separation anxiety. If the child is already in child care, parents may need to take a little extra time each day before saying goodbye. It can help to create a short goodbye ritual, perhaps involving a favorite toy. Above all, parents should try to be consistent from day to day.
12 to 24 months: Separation anxiety is most apparent at this age and can be a time when children have the most difficulty when parents leave. Children may cry or cling to their parents as they try to leave.	Parents should be understanding but firm and persistent. Once the parents have left, they should not reappear unless they intend to stay or take the child home with them.

Special Health Considerations for Child Care
❋ ❋ ❋ ❋ ❋ ❋

Health Issues	Opportunities	Concerns
Infectious diseases	❋ Training, implementing, and monitoring staff infection control practices can reduce disease rates significantly. ❋ Increased immunity to some infectious diseases may occur after the first 12 months of care.	❋ Higher rates of respiratory and diarrheal disease, especially in first year of child care. ❋ Infants in child care centers at greatest risk. ❋ Higher rates of chronic antibiotic use and antibiotic-resistant bacteria.
Injuries	❋ Safe and appropriate design and maintenance of facilities, safety rules, and adequate adult-child ratios and supervision can reduce injuries.	❋ Injuries common in child care but not more than in-home care. ❋ Most common injury occurs from falls. ❋ Playground hazards are common.
Development/behavior	❋ High-quality care has developmental, educational, and social benefits, especially for low-income children, children with history of neglect/abuse, and children with special needs.	❋ Poor-quality care may lead to inconsistent, inappropriate behavior. ❋ Infants/toddlers and children with special needs at greatest risk for neglect and abuse. ❋ Documentation issues.
Nutrition	❋ Nutrition programs (eg, Women, Infants, and Children [WIC], Child Care Food Program, and Head Start) can improve nutrition and growth, especially for low-income children.	❋ Good nutrition and toothbrushing in child care can promote dental health. ❋ Unsanitary food handling can pose a risk for food-borne disease. ❋ Inattention to food allergies can risk allergic complications. ❋ Safe and sanitary food preparation and storage can prevent food-borne illness.

Special Health Considerations for Child Care, continued

꙰ ꙰ ꙰ ꙰ ꙰ ꙰

Health Issues	Opportunities	Concerns
Child abuse and neglect	꙰ High-quality child care can provide a safe and therapeutic setting for children at risk for neglect/abuse. ꙰ Respite care, parenting education, and support through child care can reduce abuse at home. ꙰ Child care providers can recognize, report, and promote early intervention for neglect/abuse.	꙰ Child abuse/neglect may occur in child care but is not more common here than at home. ꙰ Poor-quality child care poses a risk for neglect/abuse. ꙰ Infants/toddlers and children with special needs are at greatest risk for neglect/abuse.
Staff and family health	꙰ Child care programs are required by OSHA to establish infection control and other health and safety measures. ꙰ Training, support, and work benefits can reduce health risks. ꙰ Individual and group hygiene, immunization, and use of the AAP/APHA National Standards can reduce risk of injury and illness.	꙰ Increased rate of infectious diseases, especially in first year in child care. ꙰ Risk of infectious diseases during pregnancy. ꙰ Family stress associated with balancing work and family obligations. ꙰ Back injuries aggravated by lifting children.

Infectious Diseases in Child Care Programs

Concerns About Infectious Diseases in Child Care

Children in group child care may have increased exposure to infectious diseases. Respiratory and gastrointestinal tract infections are some of the more common illnesses associated with child care settings. Infants are at particular risk because they tend to place their hands and objects in their mouths, and their hygiene and immunity are less developed. Child care providers and family members of children in child care are also at increased risk for infectious diseases.

Studies have shown that children in group child care have the following:

꙰ Increased frequency of certain infectious diseases, especially for infants in child care centers, such as: URI, otitis media, RSV, CMV, varicella, diarrheal illness, and hepatitis A. However, recent advances in medications and immunizations (eg varicella, hepatitis A) may reduce incidence of some illnesses.

꙰ Greater severity of illness, such as chronic otitis media, infant pneumonia, and invasive Hib and strep pneumoniae disease.

꙰ More frequent antibiotic use.

꙰ Increased risk for acquiring antibiotic-resistant organisms, such as Hib, strep pneumoniae, and shigella.

Other infectious diseases that are common in child care include conjunctivitis and skin infections/infestations such as impetigo, ringworm, herpes simplex, lice, and scabies.[10]

Preventing Infectious Diseases in Child Care

Caregivers, parents, and health professionals should promote the following key precautions to limit the spread of infectious diseases:

꙰ Immunizations and well care for children and adults; TB tests for adults and for children at risk.

꙰ Hand washing for children and adults after diapering/toileting, blowing noses, outdoor play, handling animals, and before handling food.

꙰ Cleaning and disinfecting toys, dining tables, kitchens, diapering/toilet areas, and cribs.

꙰ Adequate indoor ventilation and outdoor play time.

꙰ When children or adults are ill, keeping them home until they are well enough to attend, and ensuring proper medical care.

Planning for the Care of Ill Children

Parents need to understand that, even with all the prevention measures, illness is an inevitable part of childhood whether children are cared for at home or in child care. Parents need to anticipate that their child will get sick at some time. From the start, they need to have back-up child care plans for when their child is ill.

The ill child needs individualized care, nurturing, and opportunity for rest. It can be comforting for the ill child to have a familiar caregiver in a familiar setting. Parents should consider the following sick-child care options and associated costs:

※ Can the child's regular caregiver care for the sick child in the regular setting or in a sick-child area?

※ Can either of the parents stay home with the sick child? Can the parents each work a part-day schedule or work alternate days at home until the child can return to child care?

※ Is there another relative or friend that can care for the child?

※ Is there a local program that sends a caregiver to care for the sick child in the child's home or where ill children are cared for in a facility set up and staffed to care for mildly ill children? If this service is available, is the child familiar with the caregivers and the facility so using it will not cause the child additional stress?

Child Care for Children With Special Needs

Children with special needs, such as developmental disabilities and chronic illnesses, can benefit greatly from the opportunities for social contact, physical exercise, and variety of experiences in a child care program. Child care also can help the parents continue to work or pursue their education, and gain a healthy respite from the demands of caring for their child. The challenge is to find a high-quality child care program that encourages normal childhood activities and at the same time meets the child's special needs.

Children's Legal Rights to Child Care

※ *The Americans with Disabilities Act (ADA)* prohibits public and private programs from discriminating against a child based on the child's disability. It requires child care programs to make "reasonable accommodations" to provide access to facilities and services to care for the child's needs.

※ *The Individuals with Disabilities Education Act (IDEA)* states that children have a right to a free, appropriate public education in the least restrictive environment. Children with disabilities are eligible for assessment and intervention services through the local educational authority. The law requires that all children are provided with access to facilities and activities, provided with any adaptive equipment needed, and ensured confidentiality. Schools are required to involve parents in planning services for their child as documented by an Individualized Family Service Plan (IFSP) for children from birth to 3 years and their families, or an Individualized Education Plan (IEP) for children from 3 through 21 years of age.

What Parents Should Look for in a Child Care Program

1. The program should include children with and without disabilities, to the extent possible. Having normal relationships with children without disabilities can help the child with special needs feel more confident socially and helps build self-esteem. Children without disabilities also benefit by learning to develop sensitivity and respect for all people.

2. The staff should be familiar with each child's medical and developmental needs and trained to provide the special care each child requires. Staff should work with the family and the child's primary health care professional and specialists to develop an individualized health plan for the care of the child's routine and emergency needs. If the child has a chronic medical condition, staff should be trained to administer medications or perform special procedures, recognize symptoms, and access emergency medical back-up.

3. The program should have at least 1 physician consultant who is active in the development of policies and procedures.

4. The program should be flexible enough to make reasonable accommodations in facilities, activities, and equipment to adapt to the children's needs.

5. Children with disabilities should be encouraged to be as independent as their abilities allow, within the bounds of their health and safety.

References

1. Bureau of Labor Statistics. *Handbook of Labor Statistics.* Washington, DC: Bureau of Labor Statistics; 1995. Bulletin 2340

2. Casper LM. *Current Population Reports: Who's Minding Our Preschoolers?* Washington, DC: US Census Bureau; 1996. Publication P70-53. Available at: http://www.census.gov/population/www/socdemo/childcare.html. Accessed September 14, 2001

3. Heilburn S, Culkin ML. *Cost, Quality and Child Outcomes in Child Care Centers.* Denver, CO: University of Colorado; 1995

4. Galinsky E, et al. *The Study of Children in Family Child Care and Relative Care.* New York, NY: Families and Work Institute; 1994

5. American Academy of Pediatrics. *Health in Child Care: A Manual for Health Professionals.* Elk Grove Village, IL: American Academy of Pediatrics. In press

6. *The Children of the Cost, Quality, and Outcomes Study Go to School: Technical Report.* Chapel Hill, NC: Frank Porter Graham Child Development Center; 1999

7. National Institute of Child Health and Human Development. *Mother-Child Interaction and Cognitive Outcomes Associated With Early Child Care: Results of the NICHD Study.* Bethesda, MD: National Institute of Child Health and Human Development; 1997

8. Carnegie Task Force on Meeting the Needs of Young Children. *Starting Points: Meeting the Needs of Our Youngest Children.* New York, NY: Carnegie Corporation of New York; 1994

9. American Academy of Pediatrics. Part-time care for your child. In: Shelov SP, Hannemann RE, eds. *Caring for Your Baby and Young Child: Birth to Age 5.* New York, NY: Bantam Books; 1991:414–419

10. Holmes SJ, Morrow AL, Pickering LK. Child-care practices: effects of social change on the epidemiology of infectious diseases and antibiotic resistance. *Epidemiol Rev.* 1996:18

Self-
Assessment
Level One

Self-Assessment

Questions for Level One: Providing Guidance to Families About Child Care Issues

Select the *one* best answer for each question.

1. At what types of clinical visits might it be appropriate to discuss child care issues with families?
   A. Only when parents bring up the issue.
   B. At prenatal and well-baby visits only.
   C. At visits for acute and chronic conditions only.
   D. All of the above.

2. Which of the following is part of the health care professional's role in helping families make decisions about child care?
   A. Advising parents that it is best to stay home with their children.
   B. Telling families which local child care programs are the best for their child.
   C. Helping parents understand their child's development, temperament, and special needs, and considering what type of child care program might be best for their child.
   D. Telling families that child care programs care for children better than grandparents do.

3. A couple comes into your office for a prenatal visit in the 7th month of pregnancy. What would you say to initiate a conversation about child care?
   A. What are your plans for child care and what kind of child care help do you think you might need?
   B. Just focus on your pregnancy and delivery now. There is plenty of time later to think about caring for your baby.
   C. Most mothers feel guilty leaving their infants. You're not thinking about going back to work, are you?
   D. I think babies need to be with their mothers until age 2. Do you have any questions about child care?

4. The parents of a 2-month-old are starting to look for child care. A friend recommended that they take their infant to an unlicensed child care program because it is cheaper. They ask you to explain the difference between licensed and unlicensed care. How would you explain the difference?
   A. Licensed child care is by legal residents or citizens; unlicensed child care is by illegal immigrants.
   B. Licensed child care tends to be higher quality because the caregiver must have some minimum qualifications, and the facilities undergo periodic safety inspections by the licensing agency.
   C. Licensed child care is in a large child care center; unlicensed child care is in a home setting.
   D. Licensing ensures that the child care is safe, so the parents don't even need to check it out; unlicensed child care is unsafe.

5. The mother of 6-month-old twins is returning to work and starting to look for child care. She asks you to explain some of the advantages and disadvantages of in-home care, family child care, and a child care center for her infants. How would you respond?
   A. In-home care and family child care are the only options for infants; child care centers are only for preschoolers.
   B. In-home care and family child care have the advantage of keeping the infants in a home setting and limiting their exposure to other children's illnesses.
   C. Child care centers are more likely to serve the children pre-prepared frozen and canned food, which is safer than fresh food.
   D. Child care centers generally have a higher caregiver-infant ratio to allow for better supervision of infants.

6. The parents of a 3-month-old are starting to look for child care. They ask you what they should look for to find good child care for their infant. What would you advise them to look for in infant child care?
   A. Low staff-child ratio and a relationship with a primary caregiver to promote individualized attention and trust.
   B. Keeping the baby indoors all of the time to prevent illness.
   C. Frequent changes in caregiving staff to relieve stress.
   D. Diaper changing on the floor to prevent falls from the changing table.

7. The mother of a 10-month-old tells you that she needs to return to work and find child care. She is concerned because her mother-in-law told her that child care is "bad for babies." How would you respond?
   A. Maybe you shouldn't go back to work then.
   B. When babies are in child care, it interferes with bonding with their mother.
   C. If you have a good relationship with your baby, child care should not interfere. And high-quality child care can actually enhance children's development and social skills.
   D. Then ask your mother-in-law to care for your baby.

8. The parents of a 16-month-old are starting to look for child care. They ask you what they should look for to find good child care for their toddler. What would you advise them to look for in a child care program?
   A. More than 12 toddlers in a group so their child will develop social skills.
   B. Relationships and activities that nurture each child's individuality, self-confidence, self-discipline, respect for others, and social skills.
   C. A structured program that ensures toilet training by 2 years of age.
   D. Climbing equipment that is more than 2-feet high, to challenge their child's motor skills.

9. The parents of a 2½-year-old are starting to look for a preschool. They ask you what they should look for in a good preschool program for their child. What would you advise them to look for in a preschool program?
   A. New construction, no more than 10 years old.
   B. Effective use of corporal punishment.
   C. Instruction on letters and numbers to ensure preparation for kindergarten.
   D. A variety of activities and materials to stimulate their child's curiosity, creativity, and development.

10. The mother of an 8-month-old baby is returning to work and plans to have her own mother care for the baby in the grandmother's house. The grandmother is taking daily medications for arthritis and heart disease, but is fairly healthy and active. The baby is also healthy and is now crawling well and cruising on furniture. She asks what she should do to prepare her mother for caring for her baby. What would you advise?
    A. Make sure the house is "child-proofed," including storing the medications out of reach and in containers with child-resistant caps.
    B. The grandmother should not take care of the baby because she will not be able to keep up physically.
    C. The grandmother should have the baby watch television and videos for several hours a day so that she can rest.
    D. The grandmother should buy lots of baby toys and climbing equipment to provide sufficient stimulation for the baby's development.

11. The father of a 3½-year-old boy is concerned about his son starting preschool because he is "accident prone." What would you explain to him about injuries in child care and preschools?
    A. You should keep your son at home because injuries are more common in child care and preschool.
    B. Since the most common injury in child care is choking on small food, your son should be safe as long as the staff is trained in cardiopulmonary resuscitation (CPR).
    C. Since falls from climbing structures are a common cause of injuries in preschools, make sure the outdoor play structures are over grass and the indoor play structures are over carpets to cushion falls.
    D. Talk with the preschool staff about your son's behavior. Make sure the program makes a concerted effort to prevent injuries by having safe play structures over wood chips, sand, or rubber mats; safety rules; and close supervision of children.

12. A grandmother brings in her 4-year-old grandson who was in foster care and just returned to live with her and her other 2 grandchildren. He was exposed to drugs prenatally, born prematurely, and experienced neglect and abuse. He also has mild developmental delay and mild cerebral palsy. She asks you what she should do to help him with his development. What would you advise her?

    A. You don't need to worry because his developmental delay is only mild.

    B. We can wait a year or 2 until he gets into school—he'll get the help he needs then.

    C. If you enroll your grandson in Head Start or an early intervention program, he will have a complete assessment, get the therapy he needs, and have a chance to play with other children.

    D. Any preschool program would be fine for him. But don't tell them about his history or else he will be stigmatized.

13. The parents of a 6-month-old tell you that their baby is starting in family child care next month. The baby is healthy and developing well. She is breastfeeding, starting to eat solid foods, and beginning to display some separation anxiety. They ask you for some suggestions to ease the transition to child care. What would you advise?

    A. Quit breastfeeding so the baby is comfortable with bottle-feeding.

    B. Take time to explain to the caregiver about your baby's special needs, likes and dislikes, and routines.

    C. Start right away with full-day child care so the baby gets familiar with the routine.

    D. When you drop your child off in child care, sneak out so she doesn't see you leave and begin to cry.

14. A father brings his 18-month-old son for a well-child visit. He explains that his son has been in a child care center for the past 3 months. What would you say to follow up and support the child care situation?

    A. How has it been for your son in child care? How has it been for you and your wife going back to work?

    B. Are you and your wife feeling competition with your son's teacher for his affection?

    C. I bet your son's gotten sick already—they always catch things in child care.

    D. You should start working on toilet training now because child care centers like children toilet-trained by 2 years old.

15. A mother brings her 12-month-old daughter for a well-child visit. Her baby has been in family child care for a month and she is concerned that the baby cries every day when she is left there. She generally has been a happy baby and has accepted other baby-sitters. The mother says that she has not observed any signs that her baby is being abused in child care, but she worries that the "fit" might not be right with the caregiver. What would you advise her?

    A. It is normal for 12-month-olds to have separation anxiety. Leave her there and try not to worry about it—she should get over it in a couple of months.

    B. The first month in a new child care setting is always a difficult adjustment. Leave her there for another month and then reevaluate the situation.

    C. Consider calling the local child care resource and referral agency advice line to discuss your concerns. It can give you tips on talking with the caregiver about your concerns, knowing how to look for the right "fit" with the caregiver, and finding another child care situation, if necessary.

    D. Call Children's Protective Services to make a report of suspected child abuse and neglect.

16. Your 4-year-old patient is brought in with a sore throat and fever. You make the diagnosis of streptococcal pharyngitis. He attends a large, family child care home. Which of the following would be part of your treatment plan?

    A. Prescribe an appropriate antibiotic with four-times-a-day dosing because the child care provider is likely to miss doses.

    B. Tell the parent that the child should be able to return to child care for 24 hours after starting antibiotics and when the fever is gone, and when the child is acting well enough to participate in child care.

    C. Tell the parents that the child needs to stay home from child care for the week of antibiotic treatment.

    D. Advise the parent not to mention the diagnosis to the child care provider because the child will be excluded from care, and the other children already have been exposed anyway.

17. A 2-year-old child is brought into your office with a fever and rash. On examination, you make the diagnosis of chickenpox. The 2-year-old attends a child care center. What would you advise the parents about returning to child care?
    A. Their child can return to child care right away as long as he keeps the lesions covered.
    B. Their child should be kept home for a couple of days until his fever goes away and he feels better.
    C. Their child can return to child care 6 days from the start of the rash or when all the lesions are crusted over.
    D. It is not necessary to tell the center director that their child has chickenpox because the other children have already been exposed.

18. A family that you care for includes a woman and her children who are 18 months old and 3 years old. She runs a large family child care where she and an assistant care for her 2 children and 10 other children. The woman and her 2 children have been experiencing nausea, fatigue, and low-grade fever for 4 days, and she has developed jaundice. Blood tests on all 3 show hepatitis A infection. What should be included in the treatment plan and recommendations?
    A. The woman and her children should be hospitalized to prevent the spread of hepatitis A to the other children.
    B. The woman should immediately inform the child care assistant and the other families that they have been exposed to hepatitis A and to contact their health care professionals for evaluation and possible prophylactic treatment.
    C. The woman can continue to work as long as she cleans and disinfects diapering areas well, and washes her hands after toileting/diapering and before preparing food.
    D. The children can remain in child care as long as their temperature is less than 100°F.

19. Your 3-year-old patient sustained a serious burn on his hand, which is beginning to heal well. His parents ask you when he can return to his child care center. What would you advise them?
    A. He should stay home until the bandages are off and the burn is completely healed.
    B. He should go to a special sick-child care facility where nurses can care for him.
    C. He can return to his regular child care class when he is feeling comfortable and ready to participate again, and his teachers can assist him with his needs such as eating, toileting, and dressing.
    D. He should return to the 2-year-old class at his child care center where the teachers are better able to accommodate his need for assistance in eating, toileting, and dressing.

20. The father of your 4-year-old patient tells you that his wife just died in a car accident. He has kept his daughter home from preschool for the past week, but wonders when he should consider returning her to preschool. What would you advise him?
    A. He should take a 3-month leave of absence to stay home with his daughter.
    B. He should return her to her preschool when she feels ready. Her relationships with her teachers and friends can help support her through her grieving process.
    C. He should return her to her preschool but pick her up early so she doesn't see the other mothers picking up their children.
    D. He should put her in a new preschool so she won't have to explain to everyone what happened to her mother.

21. Your 3-year-old patient has a history of moderate to severe asthma. She is taking daily oral and inhaled medications, and nebulized treatment during exacerbations. She also has mild developmental delay. She attends Head Start. Which of the following should be part of your treatment plan?
    A. Recommend that she have a home-based rather than a center-based Head Start program to reduce her risk of respiratory illness and ensure that her mother is available to administer her medications.
    B. Advise the parents to give the child her asthma medication before school and after school, and not expect the Head Start staff to recognize the asthma symptoms or give her medication.
    C. Assist the Head Start health coordinator in developing a written health plan and training for teachers on the child's asthma and medications, specific triggers to avoid, signs and symptoms to watch for, and an emergency plan for responding to asthma episodes.
    D. Assure the special education staff that they do not need to be concerned about the child's asthma because it does not affect her development.

22. The parents of your 3-year-old patient are concerned that their son does not speak very clearly. They also tell you that they saw a special on television about children with attention-deficit/hyperactivity disorder and they think that their son might have it. He attends a child care center. To help in your evaluation of the child, why is it important to get the child care teacher's specific observations and assessment of the child's development, speech, and behavior?
    A. It is more convenient to get the teacher's assessment than to do a hearing test or conduct a complete developmental screening.
    B. The parents' concerns are not valid because they are too close to their child; the teacher will give a more objective opinion.
    C. The teacher has the opportunity to observe the child over an extended period of time and compare his skills and behavior to those of other children his age.
    D. Since the child has a serious developmental and behavioral problem, you will need the teacher involved for special intervention.

23. A mother brings in her 2-year-old daughter with the complaint of diarrhea for the past 3 months. In taking a history of the condition, why is it important to inquire about the girl's child care situation?
    A. It is important to assess whether her development is on track.
    B. She will not be able to get into child care until she's toilet trained.
    C. It is important to make sure the child care provider gives her enough milk and juice to keep her hydrated.
    D. If other children or staff have similar symptoms, she may have a gastrointestinal infection, such as *Giardia*, which commonly spreads among toddlers in group child care settings.

24. Understanding some of the gaps in communication between child care and health professionals, which of the following might be a good strategy for improving communication with the child care providers who care for your patients?
    A. Have your receptionist explain that you will not accept calls from child care providers because you respect families' confidentiality.
    B. Delay returning the calls from child care providers because they are usually about developmental or behavioral issues and rarely an emergency.
    C. If the child care provider excluded the child for a mild illness or communicable disease, reassure the parents that their child really should be able to attend child care.
    D. When evaluating and treating a child for an acute or a chronic condition, get the parents' consent to request caregivers' observations and to provide caregivers with key health information about the child.

Self-Assessment Levels Two and Three

Self-Assessment

Questions for Levels Two and Three: Providing Health Consultation to Child Care Programs and Advocating for Quality Child Care

Select the *one* best answer for each question.

25. How is the health consultant's relationship with a child care program different from the health care professional's relationship with patients?
    A. The child care health consultant's client is the child care program rather than the individual children and families.
    B. The child care health consultant never charges a fee.
    C. The child care health consultant does not need to be concerned about malpractice liability.
    D. The child care health consultant has no standards of care to follow.

26. You get a call from the director of a newly opened child care center. He explains that the center cares for approximately 100 infants, toddlers, and preschoolers, 15% of who have special health needs. The center also has 20 staff people. He asks you what services a health consultant could offer. Which of the following would NOT be a service offered by a health consultant?
    A. Help in developing the center's general health policies and specific protocols for the care of children with special health needs.
    B. Providing training for staff and workshops for parents on health topics such as common childhood illnesses, injury prevention, and special health needs.
    C. Conducting an on-site review to make recommendations on infection control, safety, nutrition, and developmentally appropriate practice.
    D. Suggesting that all of the families leave their current health care professionals and join your practice, to enhance continuity of care.

27. Child care health consultants should be aware of a number of legal issues that affect their practice. Which of the following is NOT a significant legal issue for child care health consultants?
    A. State child care licensing regulations, Child Abuse and Communicable Disease reporting requirements
    B. The Americans with Disabilities Act (ADA), confidentiality of health records, and parental consent for disclosure of information to staff members who need to know
    C. Clinical Laboratory Improvement Act (CLIA) requirements for licensing of clinical laboratories
    D. Occupational Safety and Health Administration (OSHA) Blood-borne Pathogens Regulations

28. What might be a good strategy to help ensure that health consultation to a child care program is effective and meets the program's needs?
    A. When you begin to work with a child care program, do a brief needs assessment to identify what the program needs your help with.
    B. When you begin to work with a child care program, explain that you have considerable expertise and tell them what they need.
    C. At your initial site visit, identify all of the problems that the program has and recommend fixing them all as soon as possible.
    D. Recommend only top-of-the-line and expensive improvements to ensure high quality.

29. A child care center director calls you to say that she is concerned that the children have had frequent gastrointestinal and respiratory illnesses. She requests that you review the center's health policy on hand washing. What would you advise?
    A. Staff and children can use moistened towelettes to clean their hands before preparing food and eating.
    B. Staff and children should wash their hands with soap and running water frequently, including after toileting/diapering and wiping noses, and before preparing food and eating.
    C. Before meals, children can wash their hands in a common bowl of soapy water.
    D. Antibacterial soap must be used and hands must be scrubbed for 30 seconds.

30. You have been asked to help a new Head Start program develop a health policy on toothbrushing. What would you advise?
    A. Each child should have his or her own labeled toothbrush.
    B. Toothpaste can be used from a communal tube and dispensed onto each child's toothbrush.
    C. Toothbrushes should be stored bristle down and covered to prevent germs from landing on them.
    D. If a toothbrush becomes contaminated, it should be disinfected in bleach or the dishwasher.

31. In visiting a large, family child care home, you observe that the backyard play area has an old metal jungle gym over grass. What would you advise?
    A. Help the caregiver check the climbing structure for safety hazards such as instability, sharp edges, protruding parts, risks for pinching/crushing and head entrapment, inadequate guard rails, and improper surfacing, according to Consumer Product Safety Commission guidelines.
    B. If the family child care serves children under 6 years of age, the climbing structure can safely be 8 feet high.
    C. Grass or ordinary gym mats are adequate impact-absorbing surfaces under a climbing structure.
    D. If you find that the climbing structure is unsafe or proper surfacing cannot be added, the caregiver should leave the structure in the yard with a sign on it warning children to keep off.

32. An infant center director calls you to explain that the center has had problems with recurrent diarrheal illness and an outbreak of hepatitis A. She asks for your assistance in preventing further illness in the center. When you visit the center, what would you be sure to observe carefully?
    A. The quantity, frequency, and nutritional quality of the foods and drinks served.
    B. The spacing between the infants' cribs in the nap room.
    C. The facility, as well as staff practices for hand washing, diapering, toileting, food/bottle preparation and storage, cleaning and disinfection of toys and surfaces, water play, and waste disposal.
    D. The developmental appropriateness of the play materials and adult supervision to support children's safe exploration of their environment.

33. When you visit a child care center, you observe staff using gloves to diaper babies. What would you advise them?
    A. The Centers for Disease Control and Prevention recommends using gloves for all diaper changes whether or not blood is present.
    B. Dirty gloves should be removed after removing the dirty diaper and wiping the baby's bottom, and before putting on the clean diaper and clothes.
    C. Latex gloves used for diapering can be reused after washing.
    D. If you use gloves for diapering, it is not necessary to wash your hands afterwards.

34. You get a call from a child care center director who is concerned that many parents bring over-the-counter cough and cold medications for their children. He asks, "What is the value of these medications? What are the risks? What should our policy be for over-the-counter medications?"
    A. Cough and cold remedies significantly improve children's symptoms and speed their recovery from colds.
    B. Cough and cold medications do not cause side effects in children.
    C. Cough and cold medications can safely be stored on the kitchen counter.
    D. Over-the-counter medications should be given only according to the instructions of the child's health care professional.

35. A family child care provider calls you to say that a child in her program has chickenpox. She asks, "When can the child return to the program? Are there any special concerns about the health of this child or other children or adults exposed to chickenpox?" How would you respond?
    A. Chickenpox is a mild childhood illness—there are no concerns about complications.
    B. The child with chickenpox can remain in child care since everyone has already been exposed.
    C. If the child with chickenpox has a fever, she should be given aspirin to make her more comfortable.
    D. If children or adults with immunosuppression, or pregnant women who never had chickenpox, are exposed to the disease, they are at risk for complications and should contact their health providers immediately.

36. A head teacher from a preschool calls to ask your advice on preventing head lice from spreading among the children in the class. What would you advise?
    A. Send a fact sheet to notify all families that their children have head lice and that they need to be treated before returning to child care.
    B. Have the entire school sprayed with insecticide to kill the lice and nits.
    C. Discard all combs, brushes, clothes, linen, bedding, and stuffed animals used by children with head lice.
    D. Check every child's head thoroughly for lice and nits. If infested, exclude them until after treatment and when they are free of nits. Recheck the children frequently.

37. A family child care provider says that some parents are concerned that their children will get sick when she takes them outdoors to play. She asks you to explain the health guidelines for outdoor play for children. How would you respond?
    A. Children should play outdoors every day, except in very extreme weather or temperatures, to develop their physical skills and reduce the spread of respiratory illnesses.
    B. Infants should not be taken outdoors or near drafts since it will cause them to catch colds.
    C. Children should not play outdoors when the ground is wet because they will catch pneumonia.
    D. Children with asthma should not play outdoors because it will trigger asthma attacks.

38. Your area has been having an unusual heat wave. A child care center director calls you to ask your recommendations on the safety of water play in child care. What would you advise?
    A. Children should not be allowed to engage in water play because it leads to an increase in illness and injuries.
    B. Water play tables and wading pools are not recommended for infants and toddlers in child care because they facilitate the spread of gastrointestinal disease. Sprinklers and individual water basins are preferable.
    C. If you put enough chlorine bleach in the water play table, children can play safely in the same water for a week.
    D. The usual adult-child ratio is adequate for supervising children in pools.

39. An infant center director calls to say that some used cribs were donated to the center. She asks you how to determine if the cribs are safe. What would you advise?
    A. A crib is safe as long as a baby has not died in it.
    B. Crib slats should be no greater than $2^{3}/_{8}$" apart to prevent head entrapment.
    C. The mattress should fit loosely, allowing at least two finger breadths on each side from the side rails.
    D. Decorative headboard cutouts and corner post extensions are safe and attractive on cribs.

40. A head teacher in an infant center calls to explain that a 15-month-old in her room has had looser and more frequent stools for the past few months. She asks, "What might be causing this? Is it contagious? Should he be excluded from child care? What should we say to the parents?" How would you respond?
    A. Infections, allergies, diet, and other rare medical conditions can cause loose and frequent stools. The parents should be informed about the changes in the child's stool patterns, advised to consult the child's health care professional, and send you a note about the child's diagnosis and treatment plan.
    B. Since loose and frequent stools are always caused by an infection, the child should be excluded from child care and only readmitted after a course of antibiotics.
    C. As long as child care programs follow universal infection control precautions, the child with diarrhea poses no risk of infection for other children and staff.
    D. The parents should be advised to stop giving their child milk and switch to drinks with electrolytes or juice.

41. A family child care provider calls you to say that she heard that the approach to fever in children has been changing. She asks you, "When a child has a fever, what does it mean? Are fevers dangerous? Does the child need to be excluded from child care? What is the best way to measure children's temperatures in child care?" How would you respond?

    A. The only accurate way to take the temperature of a child of any age is by the rectal method.

    B. Children can get elevated temperatures from illness, immunization, exercise, or hot weather. They should be excluded from child care for a temperature above 101°F orally that is accompanied by other signs and symptoms of illness.

    C. Since a child with a temperature above 99°F is highly contagious, he should be sent home from child care immediately.

    D. When a child has a temperature above 101°F, it is urgent that it be treated, so it is permissible to give acetaminophen without the consent of the parents.

42. You get a call from a director of a nursery school for 3- to 5-year olds. A father called wanting to enroll his 4-year-old son who has developmental delays and is still in diapers. The director says, "All of the children in our school are toilet trained and we are not set up to do diapering. What should we do?" What would you advise?

    A. Explain to the father that you are sorry that you will not be able to admit his son because your nursery school requires that all children be able to use the toilet independently.

    B. Explain to the father that your school curriculum cannot accommodate children with developmental delays and he will need to find another school.

    C. Explain to the father that the teachers cannot change diapers because of concerns about child abuse. But his child can attend if he comes in every day to change his son's diapers.

    D. The Americans with Disabilities Act requires schools to make reasonable accommodations to accept children with special needs, such as setting up diapering procedures and adapting the curriculum for this child.

43. A center director called you to say that he received a call from a parent who wants to enroll her 2-year-old son who has human immunodeficiency virus (HIV). The director asks you to explain the health considerations for caring for a child with HIV in child care. How would you respond?

    A. Since children with HIV are sick most of the time, they are unlikely to be able to attend the child care program consistently or benefit significantly from the program.

    B. Children with HIV can be healthy for long periods of time, and they can experience acute and chronic conditions such as recurrent infections as well as delays in growth and development.

    C. Child care programs are not required to make any special accommodations for children with HIV infection or AIDS, since it is not a disability.

    D. Since HIV can spread in a child care setting, it is recommended that staff take special precautions such as getting special immunizations and using latex gloves, masks, and gowns in caring for children with HIV.

44. A family child care provider calls you to say that a 2-year-old in her care was diagnosed with asthma. She asks you to explain what she needs to know about asthma to care for this child. How would you respond?

    A. Since asthma is hereditary, there is nothing that can be done to prevent attacks.

    B. As long as you keep the child indoors, he is not likely to have an asthma attack in your family child care.

    C. Since asthma produces coughing, as do colds and flu, it is a contagious illness and the child should be sent home.

    D. Work with the child's parents and health care professionals to identify the asthma triggers and try to remove the triggers from your family child care. Get trained to recognize the early signs and symptoms of asthma attacks, give the child's medications, and know what to do in an emergency.

45. A family child care provider calls you to say that a 3-year-old boy in her care has started being verbally and physically aggressive toward the other children. When he was going to the bathroom, she noticed that he had bruises and cuts in the shape of a belt over his buttocks and the backs of his legs. She knows that the parents have problems with alcohol abuse. What would you advise?

    A. She is legally required to make a report of suspected child abuse to the police or Children's Protective Services.

    B. She should not make a report to the police or Children's Protective Services until she has definite proof that the parents have been abusing the child.

    C. She must get the parents' permission before making a report to the police or Childrens' Protective Services.

    D. Instead of reporting the suspected child abuse, she should advise the parents to get help for their alcohol problems.

46. A center director calls you to ask what immunizations are recommended for child care staff. What would you advise?

    A. The child care program can trust that every staff person's primary care provider has given them all the necessary vaccines.

    B. Staff should be assessed for immunity to diphtheria, tetanus, polio, measles, mumps, rubella, and chickenpox. If they have not had the disease, then they should be immunized against it. Employees at risk for blood contact should be offered the hepatitis B vaccine.

    C. As long as staff were immunized as children, they do not need to worry about booster shots.

    D. There are no special vaccines that elderly staff or those with special health conditions might need.

Self-Assessment Answer Key

Self-Assessment Answer Key

Answers for Level One: Providing Guidance to Families About Child Care Issues

1. At what types of clinical visits might it be appropriate to discuss child care issues with families?

   Correct Answer

   D. All of the above.

   Health care professionals should take the opportunity to address child care issues at all types of clinical visits. When parents raise the issue of child care, it is important to address their questions and concerns. If parents do not raise the issue, however, the health care professional should ask about child care at prenatal and well-child visits as part of "anticipatory guidance." At visits for acute and chronic conditions, asking about child care can be helpful in making an assessment of the child's condition and in developing the treatment plan.

2. Which of the following is part of the health care professional's role in helping families make decisions about child care?

   Correct Answer

   C. Helping parents understand their child's development, temperament, and special needs, and considering what type of child care program might be best for their child.

   Health care professionals should ask parents about their thoughts, experiences, concerns, and questions about child care. They can help parents weigh the child care considerations for their own child and family: Should they stay at home or return to work or school? What type of child care might be best for their child's development and temperament and for their own circumstances (eg, hours, location, cost, flexibility, and reliability)? The health care professional can help parents identify what to look for in quality child care and how to find the right "fit" between their child and family and the child care setting (eg, the caregivers' style and philosophy of child rearing, activities, and amount of parent involvement). They also can refer parents to local resources such as the child care resource and referral agency.

3. A couple comes into your office for a prenatal visit in the 7th month of pregnancy. What would you say to initiate a conversation about child care?

   Correct Answer

   A. What are your plans for child care and what kind of child care help do you think you might need?

   Health care professionals should help parents anticipate child care concerns before the baby is born. Child care can be a very sensitive issue for parents—they may feel torn between a desire to stay home with their baby and a need to return to work or school; or between a desire to return to work or school and pressure from family members or friends to stay home with their baby. When health care professionals initiate a discussion with parents about child care, they should give parents the chance to discuss their thoughts, concerns, and questions without fear of being judged. Other nonjudgmental ways to open discussion of child care are: Who will help care for your baby? Are you planning to return to work or school? What are your plans for child care?

4. The parents of a 2-month-old are starting to look for child care. A friend recommended that they take their infant to an unlicensed child care program because it is cheaper. They ask you to explain the difference between licensed and unlicensed care. How would you explain the difference?

   Correct Answer

   B. Licensed child care tends to be higher quality because the caregiver must have some minimum qualifications, and the facilities undergo periodic safety inspections by the licensing agency.

   Licensed child care programs may include family child care homes, child care centers, preschools, nursery schools, and Head Start programs. Although studies have shown that licensed child care tends to be higher quality than unlicensed care, enforcement of licensing standards is imperfect and parents should not assume that all licensed child care programs are safe. Parents should be encouraged to carefully check out the quality of the child care program before enrolling their child. The health care professional can give parents a checklist (see the AAP brochure, "Child Care: What's Best for Your Family?" listed in Child Care Resources) to help them evaluate the quality of potential child care settings for their children.

5. The mother of 6-month-old twins is returning to work and starting to look for child care. She asks you to explain some of the advantages and disadvantages of in-home care, family child care, and a child care center for her infants. How would you respond?

Correct Answer

B. In-home care and family child care have the advantage of keeping the infants in a home setting and limiting their exposure to children's illnesses.

Infants can be cared for safely in in-home care, family child care, or child care centers. Each setting has advantages and disadvantages that parents need to weigh, according to the particular needs of their child and family.[1]

6. The parents of a 3-month-old child are starting to look for child care. They ask you what they should look for to find good child care for their infant. What would you advise them to look for in infant child care?

Correct Answer

A. Low staff-child ratio and a relationship with a primary caregiver to promote individualized attention and trust.

Infants are learning to trust—they need a relationship with a consistent caregiver who will understand and meet their physical and emotional needs. They should be cared for in small groups, preferably no more than 6 children, with one caregiver per 3 children. The caregiver should be warm, responsive, patient, and enjoy holding, talking, and playing with babies. The caregiver should be skilled in feeding and diapering, following proper infection control measures, and promoting infants' health and development. Infants should be exposed to fresh air and be diapered on an elevated diapering surface to prevent the spread of germs. The child care facility and equipment must be safe, and the caregiver must supervise the children adequately. The caregiver also should be committed to communicating and collaborating with parents.

7. The mother of a 10-month-old tells you that she needs to return to work and find child care. She is concerned because her mother-in-law told her that child care is "bad for babies." How would you respond?

Correct Answer

C. If you have a good relationship with your baby, child care should not interfere. And high-quality child care can actually enhance children's development and social skills.

Health care professionals should know the research on child care, dispel negative myths, and support parents in meeting their child care needs. High-quality child care has been shown to have developmental and social advantages for children. Studies have shown that children who have a good relationship with their parents and who are in high-quality child care are no more likely to experience attachment problems, injuries, or child abuse than children in home care. The one documented concern is that children, especially infants, in child care have an increased risk of infectious diseases. Good infection control practices, however, can help reduce this risk.

8. The parents of a 16-month-old are starting to look for child care. They ask you what they should look for to find good child care for their toddler. What would you advise them to look for in a child care program?

Correct Answer

B. Relationships and activities that nurture each child's individuality, self-confidence, self-discipline, respect for others, and social skills.

Toddlers are learning to explore their independence and communicate with others. They need an environment that allows them to explore safely and encourages their communication and social skills. Young toddlers should be cared for in small groups, preferably no more than 6 children, with one caregiver per 3 children. As in infant care, the caregiver should be warm, responsive, patient, and enjoy talking and playing with children. There should be a variety of activities and materials to stimulate each child's curiosity and development, and space and time for both active and quiet play. Since toddlers typically have difficulty sharing toys, there should be enough toys for all of the children. Meals and snacks should be nutritious and consist of developmentally appropriate foods with low risk of causing choking. Toilet training should proceed according to the child's interest and ability, and be coordinated with the parents' methods at home. Since toddlers actively explore their environment, it is particularly important that the child care facility and equipment be safe, and the caregiver supervise the children adequately. For children under 2, climbing equipment should be lower than 2 feet and over impact-absorbing surfacing.

9. The parents of a 2½-year-old are starting to look for a preschool. They ask you what they should look for in a good preschool program for their child. What would you advise them to look for in a preschool program?

Correct Answer

D. A variety of activities and materials to stimulate their child's curiosity, creativity, and development.

Preschoolers are learning to explore their increasing independence and mastery of self-help, motor, communication, and social skills—they need a variety of activities and materials to stimulate their curiosity, creativity, and development. They need caregivers who understand child development, set reasonable limits, and encourage children's individuality. There should be clear guidelines for effective discipline—corporal punishment should not be used. There should be space and time for active and quiet play, group and individual play, and the opportunity to choose from a variety of activities including fantasy play, looking at books, and outdoor play. Introducing children to letters and numbers may be part of the curriculum but is not necessary to ensure preparation for kindergarten. The facilities and play equipment must be safe and in good repair, whether they are new or old.

10. The mother of an 8-month-old baby is returning to work and plans to have her own mother care for the baby in the grandmother's house. The grandmother is taking daily medications for arthritis and heart disease, but is fairly healthy and active. The baby is also healthy and is now crawling well and cruising on furniture. She asks what she should do to prepare her mother for caring for the baby. What would you advise?

Correct Answer

A. Make sure the house is "child-proofed," including storing the medications out of reach and in containers with child-resistant caps.

Since the baby is beginning to crawl, cruise, and explore the environment, it is essential that the play area be made safe. "Child-proofing" should include safe storage of medications (which are common causes of child poisoning), gates to block access to stairs, electric outlet covers, and removal of small items for choking protection from the child's reach. The grandmother appears to be in adequate physical health to care for the baby. While the grandmother may need to rest during the day, she can take the opportunity to rest during the baby's naps and other quiet play activities rather than watching television. It is not necessary to buy a lot of play equipment since the infant can enjoy playing with safe household items like wooden spoons, plastic containers, and colored fabric.

11. The father of a 3½-year-old boy is concerned about his son starting preschool because he is "accident prone." What would you explain to him about injuries in child care and preschools?

Correct Answer

D. Talk with the preschool staff about your son's behavior. Make sure the program makes a concerted effort to prevent injuries by having safe play structures over wood chips, sand, or rubber mats; safety rules; and close supervision of children.

Health care professionals should encourage parents to understand their child's temperament and behavior, consider them when choosing child care, and discuss them with child care providers. While studies have shown that injuries are no more common in preschool than at home, they are a common problem for children in all settings, and the family should make sure that the preschool does all that it can to prevent injuries. The teachers should understand the child's behavior and have appropriate safety rules and supervision. The facility must also be safe. Since falls from climbing structures are a common cause of injuries in preschools, they should make sure the outdoor and indoor play structures are safe and over appropriate impact-absorbing surfaces such as wood chips, sand, or approved rubber mats—not grass or carpet.

12. A grandmother brings in her 4-year-old grandson who was in foster care and just returned to live with her and her other 2 grandchildren. He was exposed to drugs prenatally, born prematurely, and experienced neglect and abuse. He also has mild developmental delay and mild cerebral palsy. She asks you what she should do to help him with his development. What would you advise her?

Correct Answer

C. If you enroll your grandson in Head Start or an early intervention program, he will have a complete assessment, get the therapy he needs, and have a chance to play with other children.

The health care professional can play an important role in supporting families' concerns about their children's development and encouraging complete assessment and early intervention services for children with special needs. Early intervention and Head Start programs can offer significant educational and social benefits for children with special needs. For children who have experienced neglect or abuse at home, child care can provide a safe and supportive environment. It is important that the grandmother share with the program staff pertinent information about the child's medical, developmental, and social history so the program can meet the child's needs. Early intervention and Head Start programs have considerable experience with these issues and have strict policies addressing confidentiality and nondiscrimination.

13. The parents of a 6-month-old tell you that their baby is starting in family child care next month. The baby is healthy and developing well. She is breastfeeding, starting to eat solid foods, and beginning to display some separation anxiety. They ask you for some suggestions to ease the transition to child care. What would you advise?

Correct Answer

B. Take time to explain to the caregiver about your baby's special needs, likes and dislikes, and routines.

Health care professionals can help parents understand their child's development and plan for the transition to child care. From the start, parents should discuss with the caregiver their child's temperament, development, routines, and special needs—this helps the caregiver know how to care for their child, and begins to develop a relationship between the parents and caregiver. Maintaining other routines, such as breastfeeding, can enhance the baby's comfort and ease the transition to child care. It can be helpful to start child care on a part-day schedule and gradually progress to the regular schedule, if possible. Also, when leaving, it is best to say goodbye to the baby and explain that you are leaving and will pick her up later.

14. A father brings his 18-month-old son for a well-child visit. He explains that his son has been in a child care center for the past 3 months. What would you say to follow up and support the child care situation?

Correct Answer

A. How has it been for your son in child care? How has it been for you and your wife going back to work?

The transition to child care can be stressful for parents and children. It is important for health care professionals to ask about the transition and support parents' feelings. Although feeling sad or guilty about leaving the child, feeling competition with the caregiver, increased illness, and pressure to toilet train are common, the health care professional should be careful to support and not exacerbate the parents' concerns. It is important to stress that studies have shown the most important factor in a child's development is the positive relationship they have with their parents, whether or not they are in child care. Parents should be supported in the belief that they continue to be their child's primary caregiver.

15. A mother brings in her 12-month-old daughter for a well-child visit. Her baby has been in family child care for a month and she is concerned that the baby cries every day when she is left there. She generally has been a happy baby and has accepted other babysitters. The mother says that she has not observed any signs that her baby is being abused in child care, but she worries that the "fit" might not be right with the caregiver. What would you advise her?

Correct Answer

C. Consider calling the local child care resource and referral agency advice line to discuss your concerns. It can give you tips on talking with the caregiver about your concerns, knowing how to look for the right "fit" with the caregiver, and finding another child care situation, if necessary.

Health care professionals should encourage parents to continually observe and assess how the child care situation is working for them and their child. Although it is common for a 12-month-old to have separation anxiety, the parents' concerns should not be dismissed. Because the daily transition into child care can be difficult for some children, it may be advisable for the parent to visit the child care program during a nontransitional period. Parents should continue to talk to child care experts about their concerns. At this point, a report to Children's Protective Services appears unwarranted.

16. Your 4-year-old patient is brought in with a sore throat and fever. You make the diagnosis of streptococcal pharyngitis. He attends a large, family child care home. What would be part of your treatment plan?

Correct Answer

B. Tell the parent that the child should be able to return to child care 24 hours after starting antibiotics, when the fever is gone, and when the child is acting well enough to participate in child care.

When treating a child for an acute illness, the health care professional should tell the parent when the child can return to child care. The general guidelines are that children can return when the contagious period is over and when they feel well enough to participate. For strep throat, the guidelines allow the child to return to child care 24 hours after starting antibiotics and when the fever is gone. It is helpful to give the parent a note about the diagnosis and treatment plan to share with the child care provider. If an antibiotic is prescribed for an illness, it is helpful to prescribe one with less frequent dosing if possible, and ask the pharmacy to make a separate supply for home and child care, if needed.

17. A 2-year-old child is brought into your office with a fever and rash. On examination, you make the diagnosis of chickenpox. The 2-year-old attends a child care center. What would you advise the parents about returning to child care?

Correct Answer

C. Their child can return to child care 6 days from the start of the rash or when all the lesions are crusted over.

The health care professional should tell the parent when the child can return to child care. For chickenpox, the guidelines allow the child to return to child care 6 days after the start of the rash, at the end of the most contagious period. In very mild cases of chickenpox, the child can return when all of the lesions are crusted over, if that is earlier than 6 days. The parents should promptly inform the child care provider of the diagnosis in order to inform other staff, parents, and children who might be susceptible to chickenpox. Parents and caregivers should be reminded not to give aspirin to children with chickenpox because it could cause Reye syndrome.

18. A family that you care for includes a woman and children who are 18 months old and 3 years old. She runs a large family child care where she and an assistant care for her 2 children and 10 other children. The woman and her 2 children have been experiencing nausea, fatigue, and low-grade fever for 4 days, and she has developed jaundice. Blood tests on all 3 show hepatitis A infection. What should be included in the treatment plan and recommendations?

Correct Answer

B. The woman should immediately inform the child care assistant and the other families that they have been exposed to hepatitis A and to contact their health care professionals for evaluation and possible prophylactic treatment.

In addition to advising the woman to rest, drink plenty of fluids, and avoid alcohol to aid recovery from hepatitis A, the health care professional needs to advise her about measures to prevent the spread of hepatitis A to others. Close household and child care contacts, including children and family members, need to be promptly notified to consult with their health care professionals about possible prophylactic treatment. The woman should not work and her children should not attend child care until a week after the jaundice started and they are feeling better. Food preparation and toileting and diapering areas should be cleaned and disinfected thoroughly. Careful attention should be paid to washing hands after toileting/diapering and before preparing food. In addition, the health care professional should submit a communicable disease report to the public health department.

19. Your 3-year-old patient sustained a serious burn on his hand, which is beginning to heal well. His parents ask you when he can return to his child care center. What would you advise them?

    Correct Answer

    C. He can return to his regular child care class when he is feeling comfortable and ready to participate again, and his teachers can assist him with his needs such as eating, toileting, and dressing.

    During the recovery period after an injury, the health care professional should discuss with the family when the child can return to child care and what special accommodations might be needed. Returning to familiar caregivers, friends, and activities can help in the child's recovery. In most cases, as long as the child's condition is relatively stable, the child should be able to return to his regular child care. During the recovery period, the family and health care professional need to work closely with the child care staff to ensure that they are willing and able to care for the child's special needs.

20. The father of your 4-year-old patient tells you that his wife just died in a car accident. He has kept his daughter home from preschool for the past week, but wonders when he should consider returning her to preschool. What would you advise him?

    Correct Answer

    B. He should return her to her preschool when she feels ready. Her relationships with her teachers and friends can help support her through her grieving process.

    Health care professionals can offer parents advice on how to help their children cope with traumatic experiences. For a child experiencing the death of a parent, her grieving process can be supported through her relationships with trusted family members, teachers, and friends. Her father should work closely with the teachers, and possibly a mental health consultant, to understand the child's feelings and develop a plan to help her work through the process of grieving. The plan should include providing her with the opportunity to continue her old routines and play, as well as opportunities to discuss her fears and feelings of sadness, which might, for example, be triggered by seeing other mothers pick their children up from preschool.

21. Your 3-year-old patient has a history of moderate to severe asthma. She is taking daily oral and inhaled medications, and nebulized treatment during exacerbations. She also has mild developmental delay. She attends Head Start. What should be part of your treatment plan?

    Correct Answer

    C. Assist the Head Start health coordinator in developing a written health plan and training for teachers on the child's asthma and medications, specific triggers to avoid, signs and symptoms to watch for, and an emergency plan for responding to asthma episodes.

    Children with special needs, including developmental delay and asthma, can benefit from the educational and social opportunities of participating in early childhood programs such as Head Start. Early childhood programs are required by the Americans with Disabilities Act to make reasonable accommodations to facilitate the attendance of children with special needs. The health care professional should work closely with the family and Head Start staff to develop a plan to keep the child's asthma under good control, reduce illnesses and absences, and maximize her participation in the program. The child's health plan should include training for the child's teachers on asthma, triggers to avoid, signs and symptoms of an asthma attack, use of a peak flow meter, how and when to administer medications, and indications for when to call parents and emergency medical assistance. A current supply of medication and nebulizer, if necessary, should be prescribed for use at school. In addition, the health care professional should contribute to the development and review of the child's Individualized Education Plan (IEP).

22. The parents of your 3-year-old patient are concerned that their son does not speak very clearly. They also tell you that they saw a special on television about children with attention-deficit/hyperactivity disorder and they think that their son might have it. He attends a child care center. To help in your evaluation of the child, why is it important to get the child care teacher's specific observations and assessment of the child's development, speech, and behavior?

Correct Answer

C. The teacher has the opportunity to observe the child over an extended period of time and compare his skills and behavior to those of other children his age.

When parents and/or health care professionals have concerns about a child's development or behavior, the child care provider's input can be very helpful in making an assessment. The caregiver has the opportunity to observe the child's development over the full range of domains (including communication, cognitive, gross and fine motor, social, and emotional skills) and in relation to other children. The parents should be asked to explain and give specific examples of their concerns about their child's speech, development, and behavior. If an office-based hearing test and developmental screening confirm the parents' concerns, then further developmental/behavorial evaluation is warranted. If the child is found to have a problem with hearing, speech, development, or behavior, it will be important to involve the teacher in the plans for intervention.

23. A mother brings in her 2-year-old daughter with the complaint of diarrhea for the past 3 months. In taking a history of the condition, why is it important to inquire about the girl's child care situation?

Correct Answer

D. If other children or staff have similar symptoms, she may have a gastrointestinal infection, such as *Giardia*, which commonly spreads among toddlers in group child care settings.

In assessing the child's chronic diarrhea, it is important to get a full history of symptoms and exposures both at home and in child care. Since a common cause of chronic diarrhea in toddlers in group care is gastrointestinal infection (eg, *Giardia*), it is important to inquire if other child care staff or children have similar symptoms or a diagnosed infection. Since another common cause of chronic diarrhea is dietary (eg, lactose intolerance, excessive juice intake, or food allergy), it is important to inquire about food/drink history and stool patterns at child care as well as at home.

24. Understanding some of the gaps in communication between child care and health professionals, which of the following might be a good strategy for improving communication with the child care providers who care for your patients?

Correct Answer

D. When evaluating and treating a child for an acute or a chronic condition, get the parents' consent to request caregivers' observations and to provide caregivers with key health information about the child.

To best promote children's health and development, health care professionals should make an effort to develop good communication and collaboration with both parents and child care providers. The caregiver's input and collaboration are important when assessing and treating acute and chronic conditions in children. Since information about the child is confidential, it is important to get the parents' consent before communicating directly with the child care provider. It can be helpful to establish specific office procedures for receiving and responding to calls from caregivers.[2]

Answers for Levels Two and Three: Providing Health Consultation to Child Care Programs and Advocating for Quality Child Care

25. How is the health consultant's relationship with a child care program different from the health care professional's relationship with patients?

Correct Answer

A. The child care health consultant's client is the child care program rather than the individual children and families.

Since each family and staff person in the child care program should have their own primary health care professional, the health consultant should not focus on individual health issues—that is the role of the health care professional. The health consultant should focus on health issues, child care policies, implementation, and monitoring issues that apply to the children, families, and staff as a group. Examples of group health issues include infection control, injury prevention, nutrition, developmentally appropriate practices, and mental health promotion. In other respects, health consultant services may be similar to those of health care professionals, such as following standards of practice, documenting consultation, charging a fee for services provided, and safeguarding against malpractice liability.

26. You get a call from the director of a newly opened child care center. He explains that the center cares for approximately 100 infants, toddlers, and pre-schoolers, 15% of who have special health needs. The center also has 20 staff people. He asks you what services a health consultant could offer. What would NOT be a service offered by a health consultant?

Correct Answer

D. Suggesting that all of the families leave their current health care professionals and join your practice, to enhance continuity of care.

Child care health consultants can offer a broad range of services to child care programs, including developing health policies, providing health training for staff and workshops for parents, and conducting on-site reviews. In particular, child care programs that care for infants and children with special needs can benefit greatly from health consultation. Since health consultants' clients are the child care programs rather than individual children and families in the child care program, they should take care to promote and not interfere with relationships between families and their primary health care professionals. For example, health consultants can facilitate communication between center staff, families, and the children's health care professionals, when needed, and help develop protocols for the care of children with special needs in child care programs.

27. Child care health consultants should be aware of a number of legal issues that affect their practices. Which if the following is NOT a significant legal issue for child care health consultants?

Correct Answer

C. Clinical Laboratory Improvement Act (CLIA) requirements for licensing of clinical laboratories

Child care health consultants should be familiar with the laws, regulations, and standards that apply to child care programs, many of which also apply to clinical services. Health consultants can help child care programs comply with legal requirements, including state child care licensing regulations, child abuse and communicable disease reporting, the Americans with Disabilities Act (ADA), confidentiality of health records, parental consent for disclosure of health information, and Occupational Safety and Health Administration (OSHA) Blood-borne pathogens regulations.

28. What might be a good strategy to help ensure that health consultation to a child care program is effective and meets the program's needs?

Correct Answer

A. When you begin to work with a child care program, do a brief needs assessment to identify what the program needs your help with.

Health consultant services must be tailored to the needs of the individual child care program. To help address a program's needs, the health consultant should do a brief needs assessment with the director to understand the program's characteristics, health needs, and resources, and identify the program's priorities for the initial focus of health consultation. While health consultants should begin by addressing the program's concerns, they also may identify issues about which programs may not have been previously aware. It is important to prioritize the concerns and avoid overwhelming programs with too many recommendations at one time. Recommendations should be clear and simple, build on the positive things already being done, be cost effective, and easily implemented.

29. A child care center director calls you to say that she is concerned that the children have had frequent gastrointestinal and respiratory illnesses. She requests that you review the center's health policy on hand washing. What would you advise?

Correct Answer

B. Staff and children should wash their hands with soap and running water frequently, including after toileting/diapering and wiping noses, and before preparing food and eating.

All child care programs should have comprehensive health policies and health training for staff that includes hand washing. In particular, when a program has problems with frequent illnesses, it is helpful to review the health policies, inspect the facilities, and observe staff practices with hand washing, diapering/toileting, wiping noses, and food handling. Hands should be washed with soap and running water and scrubbed for at least

10 seconds. Liquid soap is preferable to bar soap because it is easier to handle; antibacterial soap is not necessary.

30. You have been asked to help a new Head Start program develop a health policy on toothbrushing. What would you advise?

Correct Answer

A. Each child should have his or her own labeled toothbrush.

Brushing teeth after lunch in early childhood programs helps prevent dental caries and teaches children important hygiene and self-care skills. Toothbrushing must be conducted properly to avoid spreading germs. Each child should have his or her own labeled toothbrush. If toothpaste is used, it should not be dispensed from a communal tube onto each child's toothbrush since this would cause cross-contamination. Instead, the toothpaste should be dispensed onto a clean piece of paper or paper cup for each child. Toothbrushes should be stored with bristles up, not touching other brushes, and allowed to air dry. If a toothbrush becomes contaminated, it should be discarded and replaced since it cannot be adequately disinfected.

31. In visiting a large, family child care home, you observe that the backyard play area has an old metal jungle gym over grass. What would you advise?

Correct Answer

A. Help the caregiver check the climbing structure for safety hazards such as instability, sharp edges, protruding parts, risks for pinching/crushing and head entrapment, inadequate guard rails, and improper surfacing, according to Consumer Product Safety Commission guidelines.

The health consultant should work with the child care provider to identify and remove safety hazards. Since falls are the most common cause of injury for children in child care, it is important to assess the safety of the climbing structure and the play area. The health consultant and caregiver can use a checklist to inspect the climbing structure for safety hazards such as instability, sharp edges, protruding parts, risks for pinching/crushing and head entrapment, inadequate guard rails, and improper surfacing. If the family child care serves children under 6 years of age, the climbing structure should be under 5½-feet high. Grass is not an adequate absorbent surface under the climbing structure

and should be replaced by 9"–12" of sand, wood mulch, or approved rubber mats. If the climbing structure is unsafe or proper surfacing cannot be added, it should be removed as soon as possible.

32. An infant center director calls you to explain that the center has had problems with recurrent diarrheal illness and an outbreak of hepatitis A. She asks for your assistance in preventing further illness in the center. When you visit the center, what would you be sure to observe carefully?

Correct Answer

C. The facility, as well as staff practices for hand washing, diapering, toileting, food/bottle preparation and storage, cleaning and disinfection of toys and surfaces, water play, and waste disposal.

Outbreaks of enteric diseases, such as diarrheal illness and hepatitis A, are common in infant centers due to frequent diaper changes and exposure to pathogens in the stool. Outbreaks are often caused by improper hand washing, diapering, toileting, food handling, and cleaning of toys. In addition, water play tables and wading pools have been found to spread enteric diseases and are not recommended for infants and toddlers. It can be helpful for the health consultant to review the health policies, inspect the facilities, and observe staff practices with hand washing, diapering, toileting, food handling, and cleaning of toys. Recommendations for preventing further illness might involve changes in health policies and/or facilities and staff training on infection control.

33. When you visit a child care center, you observe staff using gloves to diaper babies. What would you advise them?

Correct Answer

B. Dirty gloves should be removed after removing the dirty diaper and wiping the baby's bottom, and before putting on the clean diaper and clothes.

The Centers for Disease Control and Prevention recommends using gloves for contact with blood, mucous membranes, and discharges. Dirty gloves should be removed after removing the dirty diaper and wiping the baby's bottom, and before putting on the clean diaper and clothes. Contaminated gloves should be discarded in a plastic-lined, covered trash can and should not be reused. After removing gloves, hands should be washed.

34. You get a call from a child care center director who is concerned that many parents bring over-the-counter cough and cold medications for their children. He asks, "What is the value of these medications? What are the risks? What should our policy be for over-the-counter medications?"

    Correct Answer

    D. Over-the-counter medications should be given only according to the instructions of the child's health care professional.

    Cough and cold medications have not been found to significantly reduce children's symptoms or speed their recovery. In addition, the medications can cause side effects in children and, if given incorrectly, can cause overdose. Over-the-counter medications should be given only according to the instructions of the child's health care professional. They should be stored out of reach of children, not on the kitchen counter. Medications should be administered by trained staff after double checking the "5 rights" (ie, right child, right medicine, right time, right dose, right route), and documented in a written log.

35. A family child care provider calls you to say that a child in her program has chickenpox. She asks, "When can the child return to the program? Are there any special concerns about the health of this child or other children or adults exposed to chickenpox?" How would you respond?

    Correct Answer

    D. If children or adults with immunosuppression, or pregnant women who never had chickenpox are exposed to the disease, they are at risk for complications and should contact their health providers immediately.

    To reduce the spread of chickenpox to other children and adults in the child care program, the child with chickenpox should stay home until 6 days after the start of the rash or when all of the lesions are crusted over. Although chickenpox can be a mild illness for many children, it can be a serious illness for some. The lesions should be kept clean to prevent secondary bacterial infection, and the child should not be given aspirin because it could cause Reye Syndrome. Chickenpox can be life threatening for children or adults with immunosuppression (HIV/AIDS, chemotherapy, organ transplant, or steroid medication). If a pregnant woman gets chickenpox, it can infect the fetus and cause birth defects or neonatal varicella, which can be fatal. Anyone in the child care program who is immunosuppressed or pregnant should consult their health care professional immediately for possible prophylactic treatment to prevent illness. Currently, varicella vaccine is recommended for children older than 12 months of age, adolescents, and adults who have never had the illness.

36. A head teacher from a preschool calls to ask your advice on preventing head lice from spreading among the children in the class. What would you advise?

    Correct Answer

    D. Check every child's head thoroughly for lice and nits. If infested, exclude them until after treatment and when they are free of nits. Recheck the children frequently.

    Head lice is a common problem in preschools. If a coordinated approach is not initiated at school and at home, head lice can become endemic. The preschool should send a fact sheet home notifying families that their children have been exposed to head lice and what to do. All children should be checked thoroughly for head lice and nits. If they are infested, they should be treated with a pediculicide/ovicide shampoo and all of the nits should be removed. The child can return to school after treatment. At school and at home, combs and brushes should be washed; clothes, linen, bedding, and stuffed animals should be laundered; carpets and upholstery should be vacuumed; and nonwashable items should be sealed in plastic bags for 10 to 14 days. Children should be taught not to share personal care items such as combs, brushes, and hats. A child's hair and scalp should be rechecked frequently.

37. A family child care provider says that some parents are concerned that their children will get sick when she takes them outdoors to play. She asks you to explain the health guidelines for outdoor play for children. How would you respond?

    Correct Answer

    A. Children should play outdoors every day, except in extreme weather or temperatures, to develop their physical skills and reduce the spread of respiratory illnesses.

    Many families have concerns that outdoor play—cold air, drafts, and dampness—makes children sick. In fact, research shows that spending long periods of time indoors—particularly in spaces that are small, over-heated, and poorly ventilated—leads to increased illness. Exposing children to fresh air through outdoor play and opening windows helps disperse germs and reduce the spread of respiratory illnesses. Outdoor play also helps children work off energy, develop physical skills, and appreciate nature. It is recommended that children play outdoors every day except in very extreme weather or temperatures. Children who have asthma that is triggered by cold air might have outdoor activities limited on cold days.

38. Your area has been having an unusual heat wave. A child care director calls you to ask your recommendations on the safety of water play in child care. What would you advise?

Correct Answer

B. Water play tables and wading poles are not recommended for infants and toddlers in child care because they facilitate the spread of gastrointestinal disease. Sprinklers and individual water basins are preferable.

Water play can be a good learning experience, fun, and refreshing for children, especially in warm weather. However, water play tables and portable wading pools have been shown to spread disease among children, particularly infants and toddlers. Since an effective method of sanitizing water play tables and wading pools has not been determined, it is recommended instead that child care programs use sprinklers and individual water basins that are emptied, cleaned, and disinfected after each use. Pools can also be a hazard for drowning, and require a higher adult-child ratio for adequate supervision.

39. An infant center director calls to say that some used cribs were donated to the center. She asks you how to determine if the cribs are safe. What would you advise?

Correct Answer

B. Crib slats should be no greater than $2^3/_8$" apart to prevent head entrapment.

Since many older cribs do not meet current safety standards, it is important to check donated cribs thoroughly. To prevent head entrapment, crib slats should be no greater than $2^3/_8$" apart; and the mattress should fit snugly, no more than 2 finger breadths from the side rails. To prevent falls, the crib rail should be secure and at lease 36" above the mattress. To prevent clothes entanglement and strangulation, there should be no cutouts or corner posts that extend greater than $^1/_{16}$".

40. A head teacher in an infant center calls to explain that a 15-month-old in her room has had looser and more frequent stools for the past few months. She asks, "What might be causing this? Is it contagious? Should he be excluded from child care? What should we say to the parents?" How would you respond?

Correct Answer

A. Infections, allergies, diet, and other rare medical conditions can cause loose and frequent stools. The parents should be informed about the changes in the child's stool patterns, advised to consult the child's health care professional, and send you a note about the child's diagnosis and treatment plan.

It is important to note changes in children's stool patterns and report them to parents because it can be significant for the health of the child, other family members, and children and staff in child care. Since there are various possible causes of the loose and frequent stools, the child needs to be evaluated by his health care professional. The child care program should assume that the stools might be infectious, and exclude the child from child care if the stool cannot be contained in the diaper. The child can be readmitted when the diarrhea resolves, the health care professional rules out an infectious cause and another diagnosis is made, or the infection is adequately treated. Meticulous infection control needs to be followed, including hand washing, proper diapering, waste disposal, cleaning, disinfection of surfaces and toys, and food handling.

41. A family child care provider calls you to say that she heard that the approach to fever in children has been changing. She asks you, "When a child has a fever, what does it mean? Are fevers dangerous? Does the child need to be excluded from child care? What is the best way to measure children's temperatures in child care?" How would you respond?

Correct Answer

B. Children get elevated temperatures from illness, immunizations, exercise, or hot weather. They should be excluded from child care for a temperature above 101°F orally that is accompanied by other signs and symptoms of illness.

Temperatures can be taken by auxiliary, oral, ear, and rectal methods. While using the rectal method may be the most accurate, it may be uncomfortable and can pose the risk of spreading disease or injuring the child. When fever accompanies an illness, it usually helps the body fight off the disease, is not harmful, and does not need to be treated. However, if a child with a high fever is uncomfortable, removing excess clothing and blankets, offering clear liquids to drink, putting a cool compress on the forehead, or giving acetaminophen with the parents' authorization can help make the child more comfortable. The child should be sent home from child care if he has a temperature above 101°F and has other signs and symptoms of illness such as rash, vomiting, diarrhea, headache, earache, cough, or feeling too sick to participate in activities.

42. You get a call from a director of a nursery school for 3- to 5-year-olds. A father called wanting to enroll his 4-year-old son who has developmental delays and is still in diapers. The director says, "All of the children in our school are toilet trained and we are not set up to do diapering. What should we do?" What would you advise?

Correct Answer

D. The Americans with Disabilities Act requires schools to make reasonable accommodations to accept children with special needs, such as setting up diapering procedures and adapting the curriculum for this child.

The director should get more information from the father, the child's health care professional, and any other specialists working with the child about the child's special needs, intervention plan, and what the father is looking for in a school for his son. Reasonable accommodations to care for this child's diapering needs might include setting up a diaper changing table or a changing mat in a designated area away from food preparation and used just for diapering/toileting. Diapering supplies that are needed include diapers, wipes, plastic bags, latex gloves, spray bottle of disinfectant, paper towels, and a foot pedal-operated trash can. Staff should be trained and monitored in proper techniques for diapering, cleaning/disinfecting, and hand washing to prevent the spread of disease. Accommodations for the child's developmental needs might include referring the child to an early intervention program, providing additional training for staff on developmental delays, adapting the curriculum, and bringing in an aide or specialist to work with the child.

43. A center director called you to say that he received a call from a parent who wants to enroll her 2-year-old son who has human immunodeficiency virus (HIV). The director asks you to explain the health considerations for caring for a child with HIV in child care. How would you respond?

Correct Answer

B. Children with HIV can be healthy for long periods of time, and they can experience acute and chronic conditions such as recurrent infections as well as delays in growth and development.

Children with HIV infection, like all children, can benefit developmentally and socially from participating in early childhood programs. The Americans with Disabilities Act requires child care programs to make "reasonable accommodations" to care for children with disabilities, including HIV/AIDS. The symptoms of HIV are varied. Children with HIV often have no symptoms or minimal symptoms for long periods of time and usually are able to attend early childhood programs.

Children with HIV/AIDS may need accommodations to meet their needs such as early intervention services, special diets, and giving medications. Since children with HIV/AIDS may have weakened immunity, it is important to follow good infection control practices to protect them from exposure to communicable diseases, and to be alert to early signs and symptoms of illnesses.

Although there are no documented cases of HIV spreading in a child care program, the virus can spread by exposure to blood, and the same "universal" blood-borne pathogens precautions are recommended for the child with HIV as for all other children and staff—wearing latex gloves for contact with blood, cleaning up and disinfecting spills of blood, disposing of blood-contaminated items in sealed plastic bags (and sharps in special plastic containers), washing hands well, and reporting blood exposures to the supervisor and getting medical follow-up according to a written plan. (See Child Care Resources.)

44. A family child care provider calls you to say that a 2-year-old in her care was diagnosed with asthma. She asks you to explain what she needs to know about asthma to care for this child. How would you respond?

Correct Answer

D. Work with the child's parents and health care professionals to identify the asthma triggers and try to remove the triggers from your family child care. Get trained to recognize the early signs and symptoms of asthma attacks, give the child's medications, and know what to do in an emergency.

Child care providers need to work closely with parents and health care professionals to understand the child's specific asthma triggers, signs and symptoms, and medications. Child care programs can protect children with asthma from the triggers that set off attacks (eg, by following good infection control, not smoking, limiting dust, and observing the child carefully with outdoor play). Child care providers also should have written protocols and training on administering the child's medications and emergency plans for when and who to call for help. Child care providers also must comply with pertinent laws and regulations, including the Americans with Disabilities Act and their state regulations for administering medication in child care.

45. A family child care provider calls you to say that a 3-year-old boy in her care has started being verbally and physically aggressive toward the other children. When he was going to the bathroom, she noticed that he had bruises and cuts in the shape of a belt over his buttocks and the backs of his legs. She knows that the parents have problems with alcohol abuse. What would you advise?

Correct Answer

A. She is legally required to make a report of suspected child abuse to the police or Children's Protective Services.

Child care providers must be familiar with their state's requirements to report suspected child abuse—to whom the report is made, the appropriate procedures, and the necessary time frame. The report should be made promptly to protect the child's welfare. In most areas, a child abuse report can be initiated by a telephone call to the police or Children's Protective Services. Only reasonable suspicion of abuse or neglect, not definite proof, is required to make the report. The child care provider should report any information that she has from her observations of the child and anything that the child has told her about how the bruises happened.

Parent permission is not needed to make the report. However, the child care provider might feel most comfortable discussing directly with the parents her observations of the child's behavior and bruises, her concern about the welfare of the child, her obligation to report the incident, and her interest in providing support and assistance to the family, if needed.

46. A center director calls you to ask what immunizations are recommended for child care staff. What would you advise?

Correct Answer

B. Staff should be assessed for immunity to diphtheria, tetanus, polio, measles, mumps, rubella, and chickenpox. If they have not had the disease, then they should be immunized against it. Employees at risk for blood contact should be offered the hepatitis B vaccine.

Child care staff are exposed to many communicable diseases and should be up-to-date on their immunizations to prevent illness. Staff should have immunity (ie, have had the disease or immunization) to most of the same diseases as recommended for children—diphtheria, tetanus, polio, measles, mumps, rubella, chickenpox, and hepatitis B. It is particularly important for staff who are pregnant or considering pregnancy to review their immunity with their health care professional, since many of the diseases can harm the fetus. All staff should have boosters for tetanus and diphtheria vaccines every 10 years; and staff born after 1957 may need a measles vaccine. The Occupational Safety and Health Administration requires employees at risk for blood contact to be offered the hepatitis B vaccine anytime before or within 25 hours of a documented blood exposure. Staff older than 65 years of age, and those that have chronic lung, heart, kidney, or immune conditions, should get the pneumococcal vaccine and yearly influenza vaccine.

Self-Assessment Answer Key References

1. American Academy of Pediatrics. Part-time care for your child. In: Shelov SP, Hannemann RE, eds. *Caring for Your Baby and Young Child: Birth to Age 5.* New York, NY: Bantam Books; 1991:414–419

2. Dixon S. Talking to the child's physician: thoughts of the child care provider. *Young Children.* 1990;45:36–37

Child Care
Resources

Child Care Resources

Tools and Materials

American Academy of Pediatrics. *AAP Speaker's Kit on Breast-feeding Promotion and Management.* Elk Grove Village, IL: American Academy of Pediatrics. In press

American Academy of Pediatrics. *Child Care: What's Best for Your Family?* Elk Grove Village, IL: American Academy of Pediatrics; 1997

American Academy of Pediatrics. *Health in Child Care: A Manual for Health Professionals.* Elk Grove Village, IL: American Academy of Pediatrics. In press

American Academy of Pediatrics. *Moving Kids Safely in Child Care: A Child Passenger Safety Resource Kit for Child Care Providers.* Elk Grove Village, IL: American Academy of Pediatrics. In press

American Academy of Pediatrics, National Association for Education of Young Children. *Caring for Our Children: Video Series* [videotape]. Elk Grove Village, IL: American Academy of Pediatrics; 1995

American Academy of Pediatrics. Part-time care for your child. In: Shelov SP, Hannemann RE, eds. *Caring for Your Baby and Young Child: Birth to Age 5.* New York, NY: Bantam Books; 1991:414–419

American Academy of Pediatrics, Pennsylvania Chapter. *Preparing for Illness: A Joint Responsibility for Parents and Caregivers. Developed by Pennsylvania Chapter, American Academy of Pediatrics* [pamphlet]. 4th ed. Washington, DC: National Association for the Education of Young Children; 1999

American Academy of Pediatrics. *Supporting Breastfeeding Mothers as They Return to Work.* Elk Grove Village, IL: American Academy of Pediatrics; 2000

American Academy of Pediatrics. *2000 Red Book: Report of the Committee on Infectious Diseases.* Pickering LK, ed. 25th ed. Elk Grove Village, IL: American Academy of Pediatrics; 2000

American Public Health Association, American Academy of Pediatrics. *Caring for Our Children: National Health and Safety Performance Standards: Guidelines for Out-of-Home Child Care Programs.* Washington, DC: American Public Health Association; 1992

Aronson S. *Health and Safety in Child Care.* New York, NY: Harper Collins Publishers; 1991

Aronson S, Smith H, eds. *Model Child Care Health Policies.* Bryn Mawr, PA: Pennsylvania Chapter of the American Academy of Pediatrics; 1997

California Department of Education and the Center for Health Training. *Keeping Kids Healthy: Preventing and Managing Communicable Disease in Child Care.* Sacramento, CA: California Department of Education; 1994

California Department of Education and the Center for Health Training. *Keeping Kids Healthy: Preventing and Managing Communicable Disease in Child Care* [videotape]. Sacramento, CA: California Department of Education; 1994

California Department of Education and Far West Labs. *Protective Urges: Working with the Feelings of Parents and Caregivers* [videotape]. Sacramento, CA: California Department of Education; 1995

Child Care Law Center. *Caring for Children with Special Needs: the Americans with Disabilities Act and Child Care.* San Francisco, CA: Child Care Law Center; 1995

Kendrick AS, Kaufmann R, Messenger KP, eds. *Healthy Young Children: a Manual for Programs.* Washington, DC: National Association for Education of Young Children; 1995

National Resource Center for Health and Safety in Child Care. *Stepping Stones to Caring for Our Children.* Denver, CO: University of Colorado; 1997

US Department of Health and Human Services. *Training Guides for the Head Start Learning Community.* Washington, DC: US Dept of Health and Human Services; 1994–1998

US Department of Labor, Occupational Safety and Health Administration. Occupational exposure to blood-borne pathogens. *Fed Regist.* 1991;56

Organizations

Administration for Children and Families
Child Care Bureau
330 C St, SW, Room 2046
Switzer Building
Washington, DC 20447
202/690-6782
www.acf.dhhs.gov

American Academy of Pediatrics
141 Northwest Point Blvd
Elk Grove Village, IL 60009
800/433-9016
www.aap.org

American Public Health Association
1015 15th St, NW
Washington, DC 20005
202/789-5600
www.apha.org

Center for the Child Care Workforce
733 15th St, NW, Suite 1037
Washington, DC 20005-2112
202/737-7700
http://www.ccw.org

Child Care Aware
800/424-2246
http://www.cdc.gov/ncidod/hip/abc/abc.htm

Child Care Action Campaign
330 Seventh Ave, 14th Floor
New York, NY 10001
212/239-0138
http://ericps.ed.uiuc.edu/npin/reswork/workorgs/ccacamp.html

Health Resources and Services Administration
Maternal and Child Health Bureau
Infant and Early Childhood Health Branch
5600 Fishers Ln
Parklawn Building
Rockville, MD 20857
301/443-2250
http://www.os.dhhs.gov/hrsa/mchb

I Am Your Child Campaign
888/447-3400
http://www.iamyourchild.org

National Association of Child Care Resource and Referral
    Agencies (NACCRRA)
1319 F St, NW, Suite 810
Washington, DC 20004
800/424-2246
www.naccrra.net

National Association for the Education of Young Children
    (NAEYC)
1509 16th St, NW
Washington, DC 20036
800/424-2460
www.naeyc.org

National Association of Family Child Care (NAFCC)
206 Sixth Ave, Suite 900
Des Moines, IA 50309-4018
800/359-3817
http://www.nafcc.org

National Child Care Information Center (NCCIC)
243 Church St, NW, 2nd Floor
Vienna, VA 22180
800/616-2242
http://nccic.org

National Head Start Association
800/687-5044
www.hskids/tmc.org

National Resource Center for Health and Safety in Child Care
University of Colorado School of Nursing
4200 E 9th Ave, C-287
Denver, CO 80262
800/598-KIDS
www.nrc.uchsc.edu

Pennsylvania Chapter of American Academy of Pediatrics
Early Childhood Education and Linkage System (ECELS)
Building 2, Suite 307
Rosemont Business Campus
919 Conestoga Rd
Rosemont, PA 19010
610/520-9125
www.paaap.org

Zero To Three
National Center for Infants, Toddlers, and Families
734 15th St, NW, Suite 1000
Washington, DC 20005-1013
800/899-4301
www.zerotothree.org

Child Care Regulations and Legal Resources

American Academy of Pediatrics
Division of State Government Affairs
800/433-9019, ext 7666
www.aap.org

The Americans with Disabilities Act
US Department of Justice
Civil Rights Division
Disability Rights Section
http://www.usdoj.gov/crt/ada/childq%26a.htm

OSHA Requirements for Pediatric Practices
American Academy of Pediatrics
Division of Health Care Finance and Practice
800/433-9016, ext 7662
www.aap.org

Small Employers and Reasonable Accommodation
The US Equal Employment Opportunity Commission
http://www.access/gpo.gov/eeoc/facts/accommodations.html

Child Care Health and Safety Resources

Caring for Our Children
American Academy of Pediatrics, Department of Publications
800/433-9016
www.nrc.uchsc.edu

Model Child Care Health Policies
Pennsylvania Chapter of American Academy of Pediatrics
610/520-9125
www.paaap.org/frames/index.html

National Resource Center for Health and Safety in Child Care
State by State Regulations for Licensed Child Care
800/598-KIDS
http://nrc.uchsc.edu/states.html

Preparing for Illness
Pennsylvania Chapter of American Academy of Pediatrics
610/520-9125
www.paaap.org/frames/index.html

Stepping Stones to Caring for Our Children
National Resource Center for Health and Safety in Child Care
800/598-KIDS
www.nrc.uchsc.edu

Working & Breastfeeding: Can you do it? Yes you can!
National Healthy Mothers, Healthy Babies Coalition
202/863-2458
http://www.hmhb.org

The following resources have been compiled to assist pediatricians as they begin their involvement in child care activities.

1. A pediatrician's guide to child care consultation. Adapted from: the Pennsylvania Chapter of the American Academy of Pediatrics, Early Childhood Education Linkage System (ECELS) Program. 1999

2. Pennsylvania Chapter of the American Academy of Pediatrics. Child care health consultant job description. *Healthy Child Care America.* Spring 1999:11–12

3. Sample individualized health plan. Adapted from: US Department of Health and Human Services. *Training Guides for the Head Start Learning Community: Caring for Children with Chronic Conditions.* Washington, DC: US Dept of Health and Human Services; 1994–1998

4. Symptom record. Adapted from: Aronson S, Smith H, eds. *Model Child Care Health Policies.* Bryn Mawr, PA: Pennsylvania Chapter of the American Academy of Pediatrics; 1997. Adapted from: Kendrick AS, Kaufmann R, Messenger KP, eds. *Healthy Young Children: a Manual for Programs.* Washington, DC: National Association for Education of Young Children; 1995

5. Injury report form. Adapted from: Aronson S, Smith H, eds. *Model Child Care Health Policies.* Bryn Mawr, PA: Pennsylvania Chapter of the American Academy of Pediatrics; 1997

6. Medication form. Adapted from: US Department of Health and Human Services. *Training Guides for the Head Start Learning Community: Safety First: Preventing and Managing Childhood Injuries.* Washington, DC: US Dept of Health and Human Services; 1994–1998

7. *Request for Health Care Provider Evaluation.* Seattle, WA: King County Department of Public Health; 1994

8. *Care for Your Child: Making the Right Choice.* New York, NY: Child Care Action Campaign; 1996. CCAC Information Guide 13

9. Behavioral data collection sheet. Adapted from: the Pennsylvania Chapter of the American Academy of Pediatrics, Early Childhood Education Linkage System (ECELS) Program. 1997

10. Special care plan for a child with behavior problems. Adapted from: the Pennsylvania Chapter of the American Academy of Pediatrics, Early Childhood Education Linkage System (ECELS) Program. 1997

A PEDIATRICIAN'S GUIDE TO CHILD CARE CONSULTATION

Complete this form if you are using any type of child care other than care by the child's parents. Include care by others in your child's own home, in someone else's home, in a center, preschool, or after school program.

CHILD CARE AND EDUCATION FOR _____

(name of child)

When you are not with your child yourself, who is involved or who do you plan to involve with your child's care and education this year? (Include everyone to whom you give responsibility for supervising your child: family members, teachers, primary caregivers, and the child care program or school if your child is involved in this type of activity).

People:

Program or School:

QUESTIONS			
Are you looking for child care now?	**YES**	NO	**MAYBE**
Do you know how to look for quality child care?	YES	**NO**	**NOT SURE**
Is the child care you are thinking about licensed or registered with the state?	YES	NO	**NOT SURE**
Do the caregivers have training in child development, health and safety?	YES	NO	**NOT SURE**
Are the children in small groups with close adult supervision?	YES	NO	**NOT SURE**
Is more than one adult always available in case of an emergency?	YES	NO	**NOT SURE**
Is there one specific caregiver in the child care setting who has a special relationship with your child?	YES	NO	**NOT SURE**
Are you welcome to visit and see any part of the facility involved in your child's care at any time?	YES	NO	**NOT SURE**

Do the caregivers talk to you about your child every day?	YES	NO	**SOMETIMES**
Do the caregivers seem to enjoy caring for children?	YES	NO	**SOMEWHAT**
Do the children seem happy?	YES	NO	**SOMEWHAT**
Are the facilities clean and in good repair?	YES	NO	**NOT SURE**
Is there enough personal space for your child to play and rest without the other children in the group interfering ?	YES	NO	**NOT SURE**
Is there good lighting, heat, and ventilation?	YES	NO	**NOT SURE**
Does your child have opportunities for quiet and active play?	YES	NO	**NOT SURE**
Are the materials safe, interesting, and developmentally appropriate for your child?	YES	NO	**NOT SURE**
Are the active play areas equipped with cushioning materials such as wood chips or rubber mats under any equipment on which your child could climb?	YES	NO	**NOT SURE**
Do children receive nutritious snacks and meals?	YES	NO	**NOT SURE**
Do the caregivers wash their hands after toileting or diapering, before meals or food handling, after coming inside from outside, after wiping a child's nose?	YES	NO	**NOT SURE**
Do you have child care arrangements for times when your child is too sick to be in the usual child care setting?	YES	NO	**NOT SURE**
Overall, are you comfortable with your child care arrangements?	YES	NO	**SOMEWHAT**
Is there anything else you'd like to discuss about child care?	**YES**	NO	

Child Care Health Consultant Job Description

Background Information
Each child care program should have access to a child care health consultant who can provide consultation and technical assistance on child health issues. This consultant should have expertise in child health and development, and knowledge about the special needs of children in out-of-home child care settings.

Basic Functions
The child care health consultant's basic function is to prevent harm and promote optimal health in child care programs. The health consultant should seek to establish a relationship with child care providers; identify, implement, and evaluate strategies to achieve quality child care; establish basic health and safety operational guidelines and plans for the child care program and provider; and serve in a liaison capacity to other health professionals and community organizations.

The child care health consultant can be involved minimally (provide information over the telephone) or more extensively (provide advice and educational activities on-site). The health consultant should work closely with the local public health and child care resource and referral agencies and should have access to the state child care health consultant (if applicable).

Education, Expertise, and Abilities
Optimally, the child care health consultant should be a pediatrician, pediatric nurse practitioner, pediatric or community health nurse, or a health professional with expertise in mental health, nutrition, health education, oral health, environmental health, and/or emergency management. Familiarity with out-of-home child care regulations and community resources is essential. Knowledge and experience related to early brain and child development, early childhood education, and child care health and safety issues are preferred. The ability to work as a program consultant and strong written, verbal, and interpersonal communication skills are necessary.

Duties and Responsibilities
The child care health consultant can:
- Underscore the importance of a primary health care provider to serve as the "medical home" for each child.
- Ensure a system for communication among the child care provider, parent, and primary health care provider and consult when health issues arise.
- Perform on-site assessments of the child care environment and/or program operations.
- Assist child care providers in developing general policy statements and an annual plan for the child care program (eg, management of infectious diseases, fevers, and use of medications, and exclusion policies).
- Provide telephone consultation to child care providers as issues arise concerning specific policies and procedures.
- Help child care providers obtain, understand, and use information about the health status of individual children and staff.
- Educate children, their family members, and child care providers about child development, mental and physical health, safety, nutrition, and oral health issues.
- Link staff, families, and children with community health resources.
- Help identify and implement improvement plans.
- Educate and collaborate with licensing staff and policy makers to improve regulations, inspections, resources, and policies that promote safe and healthy child care.

Following are examples of specific activities of a child care health consultant:
1. Increase interactions that promote brain development.
Environment: Discuss the importance and availability of interactive play equipment.
Operations: Identify/enhance strategies to maintain adult:child ratios and recruit and retain competent staff.
2. Decrease the incidence of injuries.
Environment: Check for proper surfacing under and around playground equipment.
Operations: Ensure adequate supervision during active play.

3. Decrease the spread of infection.
Environment: Make sure adequate hand-washing equipment and supplies are provided (ie, soap, sinks, and hands-free, lidded trash cans).
Operations: Teach children and staff about proper hand-washing techniques.
4. Facilitate well-child preventive care.
Environment: Evaluate the information on the child health forms and set up a tickler system to identify children who are due for immunizations, well-child examinations, or other routine care.
Operations: Assist staff in learning how to interpret the information on the child health records as they receive them, facilitate implementation of the tickler system, and make appropriate pediatric referrals.
5. Encourage the inclusion of children with special needs.
Environment: Identify necessary changes that can be made to the physical environment to accommodate children with special needs.
Operations: Help develop an individualized treatment plan or specific guidelines for injuries or conditions of any child with special needs.

Enhancements
Administrators of larger center-based or institutional child care programs or programs serving children at increased risk may choose to identify a staff person with child health expertise or interest to serve as a point person on health issues, or as an on-site "health advocate." The health advocate can serve as a liaison between the staff and the consultant to identify and prioritize areas to be evaluated or where improvements need to occur. The consultant can educate and empower the health advocate to promote child health and safety in the child care setting on a daily basis, maximizing the effective use of available resources.

Child Care Health and Safety Resources

National Child Care Information Center
Phone: 800/616-2242
Web site: http://nccic.org

The National Child Care Information Center (NCCIC) was established by the Child Care Bureau to complement, enhance, and promote child care linkages by providing a central point for child care information. Activities include information dissemination and question-and-answer services on a wide range of child care and related topics. The NCCIC Web site features health and safety resources and includes the full text version of the Healthy Child Care America *Blueprint for Action*.

National Resource Center for Health and Safety in Child Care
Phone: 800/598-KIDS
Web site: http://nrc.uschsc.edu

The National Resource Center for Health and Safety in Child Care is located at the University of Colorado Health Sciences Center in Denver, Colorado, and is a federally funded information source on health and safety in child care settings. The Web site is a place to find the entire text of the *Caring For Our Children* and *Stepping Stones* standards for out-of-home child care programs, as well as summaries of individual states' licensing regulations.

National Training Institute for Child Care Health Consultants
Phone: 919/966-6288
Fax: 919/966-0458

The University of North Carolina School of Public Health, in partnership with the Frank Porter Graham Child Development Center, has received a 3-year grant from the Maternal and Child Health Bureau to collaborate with several organizations to develop and implement a national training program for child care health consultants. The first national train-the-trainers workshop was held in March 1999 in North Carolina.

American Academy of Pediatrics
Department of Community Pediatrics
Phone: 888/227-5409
Web site: http://www.aap.org

The American Academy of Pediatrics (AAP) Department of Community Pediatrics (DOCP) facilitates the implementation of community-based initiatives and involves pediatricians in improving access to quality health care at the community level. The DOCP frequently collaborates with the Maternal and Child Health Bureau and other organizations on projects that provide models for community action and mobilization, including the Healthy Child Care America campaign, the Breastfeeding Promotion in Pediatric Office Practices program, the Medical Home Program for Children with Special Needs, the Healthy Tomorrows Partnership for Children Program, and the Community Access to Child Health (CATCH) program. The vision of CATCH is that every child has a medical home and other needed services to reach optimal health and well-being. The Academy strives to include these concepts as a visible part of the Healthy Child Care America campaign. Through the department, training, technical assistance and educational materials are available to assist those interested in promoting access to child health and implementing community-based initiatives.

Caring for Our Children: National Health and Safety Performance Standards: Guidelines for Out-of-Home Child Care Programs, the *Caring for Our Children* manual and video

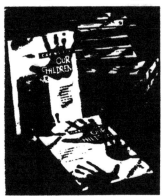

series; and *the Model Child Care Health Policies* booklet (developed by the AAP Pennsylvania chapter); and the *Safe Active Play* video are available by contacting the AAP Division of Publications at 800/433-9016, ext 5898.

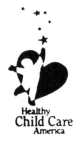

Healthy
Child Care
America

For more information on the Healthy Child Care America campaign, call 888/227-5409 or e-mail childcare@aap.org.

Sample Individualized Health Plan

ROUTINE CARE

Today's Date: _____ Review No Later Than: _____

Child: _____ Birth Date: _____

Parent(s) or Guardian(s): _____ Phone #: _____

Primary Health Care Provider: _____ Phone #: _____

Diagnosis: 1. _____ 2. _____ 3. _____

REGULARLY-SCHEDULED MEDICATIONS

Medication	Schedule (When)	Dose (How Much)	Route (How)	Possible Side Effects

Describe accommodations the child
needs in daily activities:

Check whether accommodations
needed at: HOME   SCHOOL

• Diet or Feeding: _____   _____

• Classroom Activities: _____   _____

• Naptime/Sleeping: _____   _____

• Toileting: _____   _____

• Outdoor Activities/Field Trips: _____   _____

• Transportation: _____   _____

• Other: _____   _____

Sample Individualized Health Plan *(continued)*

EMERGENCY CARE

Child: _____ **Birth Date:** _____

Parent(s) or Guardian(s): _____ **Phone #:** _____

Primary Health Care Provider: _____ **Phone #:** _____

Diagnosis: 1. _____   2. _____   3. _____

CALL PARENTS FOR:

> **While waiting for parent(s) or medical help to arrive:**

GIVE AS NEEDED OR EMERGENCY MEDICATION FOR:

Medication	Schedule (When)	Dose (How Much)	Route (How)	Possible Side Effects

GET MEDICAL ATTENTION FOR: **CALL 911 (Emergency Medical Services) FOR:**

I have helped develop this health plan. I understand it and will try my best to follow the plan. I will communicate any changes in the child's condition or treatment. Plan completed: _____ (date). Plan will be updated on or before: _____ (date).

Parent(s) or Guardian(s): _____

Staff Name(s) & Title(s): _____

Health Care Provider Name(s) & Title(s): _____

Other: _____

Symptom Record

Child's name: _____ **Date:** _____

MAIN SYMPTOM _____

When it began _____ How long it has lasted_____

How much _____ How often _____

Staying constant, getting better or worse? _____

OTHER SYMPTOMS: Complaints _____
General appearance *(eg, comfort, mood, behavior, activity level, appetite)*

CIRCLE THE SYMPTOMS:

Breathing: *coughing*   *wheezing*   *breathing fast*   *difficulty breathing*   *other* _____

Skin: *pale*   *flushed*   *rash*   *sores*   *swelling*   *bruises*   *itchiness*   *other* _____

Vomiting: *(# times)* _____ Diarrhea *(# times)* _____ Urine _____

Eyes: *pink/red*   *watery*   *discharge*   *crusty*   *swollen*   *other* _____

Nose: *congested*   *runny*   *other* _____

Ears: *pulling at ears*   *discharge*   *other* _____

Mouth: *sores*   *drooling*   *difficulty swallowing*   *other* _____

Odors: *(eg, breath, stool)* _____

Temperature: _____ *(axillary   oral   rectal   other* _____)

WHAT HAS BEEN DONE: Comfort _____ Rest _____

Liquids *(name, amount, time)* _____ Food *(name, amount, time)* _____

Medications *(name, amount, time)* _____

Emergency measures _____

Who was called and when *(eg, parent/guardian, emergency contact person, health consultant, child's health provider, emergency medical services)*

_____

Signature _____

Adapted from: *Model Child Care Health Policies,* American Academy of Pediatrics, Pennsylvania Chapter, 1997, and *Healthy Young Children: A Manual for Programs,* National Association for the Education of Young Children, 1995.

Injury Report Form

Name of Program: _____ **Phone:** _____

Address of Facility: _____

Child's Name: _____ **Sex:** M F **Birth Date:** __/__/__ **Incident Date:** __/__/__

Time of Incident: ___:___ AM/PM **Witness:** _____

Location of Incident: ☐ playground ☐ classroom ☐ bathroom ☐ hall ☐ kitchen ☐ doorway ☐ office
☐ dining room ☐ large muscle room or gym ☐ stairway ☐ unknown ☐ other (specify):

Equipment/Product Involved: ☐ climber ☐ slide ☐ swing ☐ playground surface ☐ sandbox ☐ trike/bike
☐ hand toy (specify): _____ ☐ other equipment (specify): _____

Cause of Injury: ☐ fall to surface; estimated height of fall _____ feet; type of surface: _____
☐ fall from running/tripping ☐ bitten by child ☐ hit or pushed by child ☐ injured by object: _____
☐ eating or choking ☐ insect sting/bite ☐ animal bite ☐ exposure to cold ☐ motor vehicle
☐ other (specify): _____

Parts of Body Injured: ☐ eye ☐ ear ☐ nose ☐ mouth ☐ tooth ☐ other part of face ☐ other part of head
☐ neck ☐ arm/wrist/hand ☐ leg/ankle/foot ☐ trunk ☐ other (specify): _____

Type of Injury: ☐ cut ☐ bruise or swelling ☐ puncture ☐ scrape ☐ broken bone or dislocation ☐ sprain
☐ crushing injury ☐ burn ☐ loss of consciousness ☐ unknown ☐ other (specify): _____

First Aid Given at the Facility: ☐ comfort ☐ pressure ☐ elevation ☐ ice ☐ cleaned wound
☐ antiseptic ☐ bandage ☐ rest ☐ other (specify): _____

Who was Contacted at What Time: ☐ parents at ___:___ AM/PM ☐ health care provider at ___:___ AM/PM
☐ emergency contact person at ___:___ AM/PM ☐ emergency medical services at ___:___ AM/PM
☐ other (specify): _____ at ___:___ AM/PM

Treatment Provided by: _____
☐ no doctor's or dentist's treatment required ☐ treatment as an outpatient (eg, office or emergency room)
☐ hospitalized (overnight) # of days: _____ ☐ other (specify): _____

Follow-up Plan for Care of the Child: _____

Corrective Action Needed to Prevent Reoccurrence: _____

Name of Official/Agency Notified: _____ **Date:** _____

Signature of Staff Member: _____ **Date:** _____

Signature of Parent: _____ **Date:** _____

Adapted with permission from: Pennsylvania Chapter of the American
Academy of Pediatrics (June 1997) *Model Child Care Health Policies.*

MEDICATION

Today's Date:

Child _____ **Birth Date:** _____

Parent(s) or Guardian(s): _____ **Phone #:** _____

Primary Health Care Provider: _____ **Phone #:** _____

DIAGNOSIS: 1. _____ 2. _____ 3. _____

Medication	Schedule (When)	Dose (How Much)	Route (How)	Possible Side Effects

Adapted with permission from: Pennsylvania Chapter of the American Academy of Pediatrics (June 1997) *Model Child Care Health Policies.*

REQUEST FOR HEALTH CARE PROVIDER EVALUATION

PROGRAM:	CONTACT PERSON:	TELEPHONE NUMBER:	DATE:

TO BE COMPLETED BY CHILD CARE PROVIDER

(CHILD'S NAME) _____ (DATE OF BIRTH) _____

The following signs and / or symptoms have been noted:

☐ Cold, runny nose   ☐ Fever _____   ☐ Rash

☐ Cough / Wheezing   ☐ Yellow skin or eyes   ☐ Skin Sores

☐ Dark Urine   ☐ White or Grey Stool   ☐ Sore throat

☐ Diarrhea   ☐ Mouth Sores   ☐ Vomiting

☐ Eye drainage   ☐ Pain

☐ Other concerns in our daily health observation:

_____

☐ Cases of _____ have recently been reported in other children
attending our program.

HEALTH CARE PROVIDER, PLEASE EVALUATE THIS CHILD AND COMPLETE THIS FORM.

DIAGNOSIS: ☐ Communicable   If this is communicable, what is the name of the disease?_____

           ☐ Not communicable

TREATMENT: ☐ No treatment necessary

           ☐ Treatment recommended _____

           ☐ Duration _____

CAN CHILD RETURN TO CHILD CARE NOW?

☐ Yes   ☐ No   If "No" when can the child return?_____

COMMENTS:

HEALTH CARE PROVIDER SIGNATURE:	PHONE NUMBER:	DATE:

Parent or guardian, please return this completed form to the child care program when the child returns.

Seattle-King County Department of Public Health
March 1994

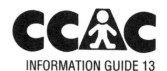

Care For Your Child: Making the Right Choice

INFORMATION GUIDE 13

CHILD CARE ACTION CAMPAIGN • 330 Seventh Avenue, 17th Floor, New York, NY 10001 (212) 239-0138

Parents today attempt to solve their child care needs in many ways. Some parents arrange to have family members care for younger children. Other parents choose an arrangement available in the community. The common types of care are:

CARE WITHIN THE FAMILY

Close to half of all working parents with children under age five use this type of care, which includes:

• Arranging work hours so that one parent is always home;

• Relying on a relative, older sibling or very close friend; or

• Combinations of these arrangements.

CARE IN THE COMMUNITY

Used by over 7 million families. This includes:

• **In-home care.** A trained child care provider, nanny or babysitter comes to the child's home. This is a very expensive solution for full-time care since one family pays the caregiver's entire salary.

• **Shared care.** Several families employ a caregiver to care for all of their children in one home.

• **Family child care.** Several children are cared for in the provider's home.

• **Group child care homes.** A provider cares for a specified number of children in his/her home with assistance. Additional adults are employed as indicated by state requirements for staff/child ratios for the particular ages of the children receiving care.

• **Child care centers.** A center provides care for groups of children in a facility designed for children. It is licensed by the state and must meet state standards for child/staff ratios, teacher training and group size. Centers are operated by for-profit and not-for-profit entities. About one third of all child care centers in the U.S. are housed in church or synagogue buildings.

• **Mixed arrangements.** Typically, parents make more than one arrangement for their child, combining part-day programs with a home-based care.

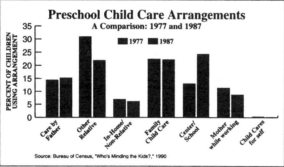

Preschool Child Care Arrangements
A Comparison: 1977 and 1987

Source: Bureau of Census, "Who's Minding the Kids?," 1990

Child care centers and family day care programs are also used by parents who do not work outside the home because of the educational and social benefits such centers can offer children.

CHOOSING AN ARRANGEMENT

Child care decisions are among the most important that families face. They should be made carefully. Use as many resources as are available to you to find the quality care you need. Here are some factors that you should consider in choosing the best arrangement for you and your child:

1. Licensing. State licensing requirements generally assure the basic health and safety of a facility but may not guarantee the quality you are looking for. Be sure to check your state's

licensing standards and ask any prospective care facility if it complies. If the child care facility is not licensed, find out why.

2. Quality. Some high quality center-based programs have been accredited by the National Association for the Education of Young Children (NAEYC). Ask about a center's accreditation. Even if it has not been accredited, some key elements of quality to look for include: staff structure; staff training; interactions between children and providers; cleanliness; safety and adequate, age-appropriate equipment. Visit the program. Talk to other parents; their experiences can help you learn what to look for.

3. Group Size and Ratios. The most important factors contributing to the quality of a child care program are group size; the ratio of staff to children and staff training and experience. Studies show that children benefit the most, both socially and developmentally from being in smaller child care groups; smaller sizes allow for more direct social interaction between children and caregivers. Although state regulations vary, the following are optimal staff to child ratios that ensure that children will receive enough individual attention:

Family Day Care – 1 adult to 5 children, including the caregiver's own (no more than two infants under one year)

Day Care Centers – 1 adult to 3-4 infants or toddlers

1 adult to 4-6 two year olds

1 adult to 7-8 three year olds

1 adult to 8-9 four year olds

1 adult to 8-10 five year olds

1 adult to 10-12 after-school children

The total size of the group should be

no more than two times the staff/child ratio. For example, infants should be in a group with no more than eight children.

4. Training. Because there are no consistent standards for child care staff training, child care workers' experience and education vary widely. Qualified staff may have college degrees in early childhood education or a Child Development Associates credential. If the caregivers at a prospective facility do not have such formal training, ask if the program provides in-service training for staff. Whatever their formal training, you will want to observe the staff as they interact with the children under their care. Firsthand observation is the most reliable means of assessing a caregiver's ability to care for your child. Ask about staff turnover; low wages for caregivers are the main reason for extremely high turnover in the child care field, and such turnover negatively affects the quality of care.

5. Adult-to-Child and Child-to-Child Interactions. Watch carefully to see if the children are busy, happy and absorbed in their activities. Observe the adults. Are they interested, loving and actively involved with the children?

6. Cleanliness. The spread of infectious diseases can be controlled by cleanliness. Watch to see if teachers or other adults wash their hands frequently, especially after diaper changing. Do children wash before eating and after going to the toilet? Are the facilities, toys and equipment cleaned regularly?

7. Play Equipment. A variety of interesting play materials and equipment can help your child achieve physical, social and intellectual growth. In addition, it's important that each age group be provided with enough age-appropriate play materials. For example, jigsaw puzzles and crayons may be fine for preschoolers but are inappropriate for infants. Keeping this in mind,

look for play materials such as books, blocks of all sizes, wheel toys, balls, puzzles, plants, science materials, small manipulative materials, musical toys, housekeeping toys, and large climbing equipment appropriate to the age group.

8. Safety and Emergency Procedures. There should be an emergency plan clearly posted near the telephone. This should include telephone numbers for a doctor, ambulance, fire department, police, etc. Smoke detectors should be installed and fire extinguishers must be readily available and in working order. Although it is difficult to think about, accidents do happen to children, whether they are at home or in child care. Staff should be trained to deal with emergencies.

9. Price of Care. Fees for child care services vary greatly. The price for family day care ranges from $10 to $120 per child, per week. In centers, care for infants (0-2 years) is usually the most expensive, costing between $20 and $200 per week. Rates range from $25 to $170 per week for preschoolers. In-home caregivers must be paid at least the minimum wage, and parents are responsible for Social Security and other taxes. Despite the high fees, child care providers are among the lowest paid in the United States, earning an average $5.35 per hour. The federal government and some state governments offer tax credit programs to help parents pay for child care; some employers also help out with child care expenses. (CCAC Information Guides #16, *"How to Use the Federal Child Care Tax Credit,"* and #9, *"Speaking with Your Employer About Child Care Assistance,"* provide further details.)

10. Location. Transportation and location, like costs, determine whether a program is within a family's reach. When possible, choose child care close to your home or work. Sometimes a center en route to work, near the school that an older child attends or near a relative can be a good choice as well.

RESOURCES TO HELP PARENTS FIND CHILD CARE
RESOURCE AND REFERRAL AGENCIES

Resource and Referral (R&R) agencies educate parents about the types of care that are available. They will give you a list of child care programs in your area, and pointers about what to look for when evaluating a potential caregiver. R&R's provide an important community service as well. They may recruit and train new providers, help start new child care programs, and sponsor parent education seminars. Some gather data on the need for child care services, and work toward improving the quality of a community's child care supply. Many R&R's get involved in the public policy debate on child care. For information about the R&R agency in your area, contact:

National Association of Child Care Resource and Referral Agencies (NACCRRA.) 2116 Campus Drive SE, Rochester, MN 55904, (507) 287-2220

Check also with your state's Department of Human Services and in the Yellow Pages under "Child Care." Some corporations offer resource and referral services for employees; check with your company's Human Resources department.

Licensing Agencies. States and some cities license and regulate child care providers. Usually the licensing office is in a social service or health department; sometimes it is in a children's agency. When you call the agency, be sure to ask about the different types of child care available – child care centers or licensed family day group homes. (CCAC Information Guide #28, *"Current State Day Care Licensing Offices,"* provides a list.)

Civic Organizations. Groups such as the National Council of Jewish Women (NCJW), the National Organization for Women (NOW), the Junior League, the Business and Professional

Women's Association, and the United Way may also know about child care in your community. While these organizations may have information about a wide range of services, they probably will not be able to advise you on how to choose a facility. They may, however, be able to steer you to someone who does know.

Yellow Pages. Child care providers may be listed here, although not all choose to be listed. Family day care, for example, is not well represented in the Yellow Pages. Look under: "Child Care," "Day Care," "Day Nurseries," and "Nursery Schools."

Community Bulletin Boards. Some child care programs and providers advertise their services by placing notices on these boards. You can find bulletin boards in shopping centers, laundromats, libraries, and other public places.

Local YWCAs, YMCAs, YWHAs, and YMHAs. "Y" staff may be familiar with the different child care programs in your community. Many Y's even run their own child care programs, nursery schools or after-school programs.

Churches and Synagogues. Many churches and synagogues house child care centers. They may also be familiar with other programs in your area.

Parent Support Groups and Parenting Newspapers. Parents in many communities have started parent support groups and parenting newsletters. Both give parents emotional support as well as specific advice about child development and child care. Talk to other parents to see if there is a parenting group or newspaper in your area. Check with teachers, your local churches and synagogues, and community-based organizations too.

Newspaper Advertisements. Both parents and providers try to reach one another by placing ads in the classified section of the newspaper. Your community paper may be an especially good place to find programs and providers.

Local Colleges. Colleges that offer degrees in early childhood education may run laboratory child care centers. These centers usually employ a full-time professional staff and use students on a rotating basis. Colleges may also be able to refer you to high-quality child care programs in your area. Find out where they send their own early childhood education students for training. You may also be able to find an in-home caregiver or a part-time babysitter through the college. Check bulletin boards – students sometimes offer their services there – or place an ad in the school newspaper.

Pediatricians. Because of their regular contact with other parents and children, pediatricians may know of child care programs and providers.

Child Care Employment Agencies. These agencies help you find in-home care. Check in the Yellow Pages under "Babysitting Services" or "Child Care," or ask a local R&R.

Once you've compiled a list of child care facilities in your area, call each of the programs or providers. Find out where there are vacancies, what kinds of programs are offered, and which ones you can afford. Ask about waiting lists, hours, holiday/vacation schedules, references and licensing. After a preliminary telephone conversation, set up appointments with those that sound promising. It is absolutely essential that you visit and evaluate any child care facility that you are seriously considering for your child.

ENSURING GOOD CHILD CARE

The best insurance you have that your child care arrangement will be best for you and your child is **your own thorough observation.**

• Before and after choosing a child care program, visit the facility, get to know the other parents, and discuss your child's behavior and development with the caregivers.

• Observe the caregivers' interactions with the children and decide for yourself whether your child is receiving the loving care you want.

• Never enroll your child in a center or family day care home where you are not welcome to drop in unannounced.

• Pay attention to how your child and other children respond to the program and staff. The quality can vary greatly over time due to staff turnover or other factors.

• Take note if your child continues to be unhappy after some time in child care, suddenly becomes unhappy after having gotten adjusted, talks about being afraid or disliking child care or a particular caregiver, or has injuries that the caregiver cannot adequately explain. These are warning signs that are cause for thorough investigation of the child care facility and discussion with staff.

CCAC Information Guide #19, *"Finding Good Child Care"*; and #20, *"Who's Caring for Your Kids? What Every Parent Should Know About Child Care Providers,"* are also helpful. Additional Resources include:

"Going to Work? Choosing Care for Infants and Toddlers" by Joan Bergstrom and Linda Joy available from Joan Bergstrom, 303 Marsh Street, Belmont, MA 02178 (price $2.50)

"The Parent's Guide to Day Care," by Jo Ann Miller and Susan Weissman Bantam Books, New York, 1986. Child care resource and referral agencies also have guidance material that can be helpful as you look for child care in your community.

"Child Care Resource and Referral: 1989 Survey Findings," available from the National Association of Child Care Resource and Referral Agencies 2116 Campus Drive SE Rochester, MN 55904 (price $5 member, $15 non-member)

BEHAVIORAL DATA COLLECTION SHEET

This sheet is intended to be used by caregivers to document a child's behavior that is of concern to them. The behavior may warrant evaluation by a health care provider, discussion with parents, and/or consultation with other professionals.

Child's name: _____ Date: _____

1. Describe behavior observed: (see below for some descriptions)
   _____

2. Behavior noted from: _____ to _____
                                 (time)   *(time)*

3. During that time, how often did the child engage in the behavior (eg, once, 2–5 times, 6–10 times, 11–25 times, >25 times, >100 times) _____

4. What activity(ies) was the child involved in when the behavior occurred? (eg, Was the child involved in a task? Was the child alone? Had the child been denied access to a special toy, food, or activity?)
   _____

5. Where did the behavior occur? _____

6. Who was around the child when the behavior began? (list staff, children, parents, others)
   _____

7. Did the behavior seem to occur for no reason? Did it seem affected by changes in the environment?
   _____

8. Did the child sustain any self-injury? Describe. _____

9. Did the child cause property damage or injury to others? Describe. _____
   _____

10. How did caregiver respond to the child's behavior? If others were involved, how did they respond?
    _____

11. What did the child do after caregiver's response? _____

12. Have parents reported any unusual situation or experience the child had since attending child care? _____

Child care facility name: _____

Name of caregiver completing this form: _____

Behaviors can include:
- *repetitive, self-stimulating acts*
- *self-injurious behavior (SIB) such as head banging, self-biting, eye-poking, pica (eating nonfood items), pulling out own hair*
- *aggression/injury to others*
- *disruption such as throwing things, banging on walls, stripping*
- *agitation such as screaming, pacing, hyperventilating*
- *refusing to eat/speak; acting detached / withdrawn*
- *others*

Check a child's developmental stage before labeling a behavior a problem. For example, it is not unusual for a 12-month-old to eat nonfood items, nor is it unusual for an 18-month-old to throw things. Also note how regularly the child exhibits the behavior. An isolated behavior is usually not a problem.

S. Bradley, JD, RN,C — PA Chapter of the American Academy of Pediatrics
reviewed by J. Hampel, PhD and R. Zager, MD

SPECIAL CARE PLAN FOR A CHILD WITH BEHAVIOR PROBLEMS

*This sheet is intended to be used by health care providers and other professionals
to formulate a plan of care for children with severe behavior problems
that parents and child care providers can agree upon and follow consistently.*

Part A: To be completed by parent/custodian

Child's name:_____ Date of birth: _____

Parent name(s): _____

Parent emergency numbers: _____

Child care facility/school name:_____ Phone: _____

Health care provider's name: _____ Phone: _____

Other specialist's name/title:_____ Phone: _____

Part B: To be completed by health care provider, pediatric psychiatrist, child psychologist, or other specialist

1. Identify/describe behavior problem: _____

2. Possible causes/purposes for this type of behavior: *(Circle all that apply.)*

    medical condition _____   tension release

                      (Specify.)   developmental disorder

    attention-getting mechanism   neurochemical imbalance

    gain access to restricted items/activities   frustration

    escape performance of task   poor self-regulation skills

    psychiatric disorder _____   other: _____

                      (Specify.)

3. Accommodations needed by this child: _____

    _____

4. List any precipitating factors known to trigger behavior: _____

    _____

5. How should caregiver react when behavior begins? *(Circle all that apply.)*

    ignore behavior   physical guidance (including hand-over-hand)

    avoid eye contact/conversation   model behavior

    request desired behavior   use diversion/distraction

    use helmet*   use substitution

    use pillow or other device to block self-injurious behavior (SIB)*

    other: _____

    _____

    *directions for use described by health professional in Part D.

6. List any special equipment this child needs: _____

    _____

7. List any medications this child receives:

   Name of medication: _____   Name of medication: _____

   Dose: _____   Dose: _____

   When to use: _____   When to use: _____

   Side effects: _____   Side effects: _____

   _____   _____

   Special instructions: _____   Special instructions: _____

   _____   _____

8. Training staff need to care for this child: _____

   _____

9. List any other instructions for caregivers: _____

   _____

Part C: Signatures

Date to review/update this plan: _____

Health care provider's signature: _____   Date: _____

Other specialist's signature: _____   Date: _____

Parent signature(s): _____   Date: _____

_____   Date: _____

Child care/school director: _____   Date: _____

Primary caregiver signature: _____   Date: _____

Part D: To be completed by health care provider, pediatric psychiatrist, child psychologist, or other specialist

Directions for use of helmet, pillow, or other behavior protocol: _____

_____

_____

_____

_____

_____

_____

_____

S. Bradley, JD, RN,C — PA Chapter of the American Academy of Pediatrics
reviewed by J. Hampel, PhD and R. Zager, MD
April 1997